AF614763

Pulmonary Emphysema - Recent Updates

Edited by Kian Chung Ong

Published in London, United Kingdom

Pulmonary Emphysema - Recent Updates
http://dx.doi.org/10.5772/intechopen.1005625
Edited by Kian Chung Ong

Contributors
Alexandru Mihai Cornea, Alina Ligia Cornea, Balachandar Selvakumar, Diana Parau, Earnest Arul, Isidora Simonovic, Kian Chung Ong, Lana Kourieh, Ola Arab, Peter Riddell, Radmila Dmitrovic, Seamus Linnane

First published in London, United Kingdom, 2024 by IntechOpen
IntechOpen is the global imprint of INTECHOPEN LIMITED, registered in England and Wales, registration number: 11086078, 167-169 Great Portland Street, London, W1W 5PF, United Kingdom

British Library Cataloguing-in-Publication Data
A catalogue record for this book is available from the British Library

Additional hard and PDF copies can be obtained from orders@intechopen.com

Pulmonary Emphysema - Recent Updates
Edited by Kian Chung Ong
p. cm.
Print ISBN 978-0-85466-329-3
Online ISBN 978-0-85466-328-6
eBook (PDF) ISBN 978-0-85466-330-9

For EU product safety concerns:
IN TECH d.o.o., Prolaz Marije Krucifikse Kozulić 3, 51000 Rijeka, Croatia,
info@intechopen.com or visit our website at intechopen.com.

Meet the editor

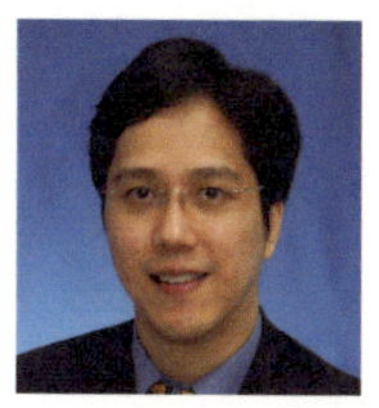

Dr. Kian Chung Ong is a specialist in respiratory and intensive care medicine with 25 years of clinical experience. He is presently the medical director of the Chestmed Clinic, Mount Elizabeth Medical Centre, Singapore. Dr. Ong has authored more than 50 scientific papers and 12 book chapters and is the editor of five open-access textbooks apropos to respiratory medicine. He is a member of the Global Initiative for Chronic Obstructive Lung Disease (GOLD) Assembly since its establishment in 2000. He is also the founder and current president of the Chronic Obstructive Pulmonary Disease Association (Singapore). Beyond meeting the clinical demands of private specialist practice, Dr. Ong is committed to conducting translational research in lung disease with tertiary academic institutions in Singapore.

Contents

Preface

The title of this textbook may require some explication. First, pulmonary emphysema has been, for several decades now, subsumed under the umbrella term "chronic obstructive pulmonary disease", better known by the acronym COPD. The historical journey in the development of the term "COPD" is briefly retraced in the introductory chapter. The reasons for retaining the term "emphysema" for this textbook are not just sentimental but specific, namely, to limit the subject matter to a narrower phenotype and pathology. Second, "recent updates" is a deliberate double emphasis. The reader can be assured that contributors to the current volume aim to disseminate information and discuss issues that are au courant. The introductory chapter addresses the latest major updates in the Global Initiative for Obstructive Lung Disease (GOLD) Strategy for Prevention, Diagnosis and Management of COPD. In particular, the recently adopted changes to the definition, nomenclature, and taxonomy (classification) of COPD are elaborated and the rationale behind the major revisions is explored. In the realm of basic scientific research, the central pathophysiological role of macrophages in pulmonary emphysema is expertly summarized in the second chapter. Keen understanding and further research in this area may potentiate the development of novel therapeutic strategies for reducing lung damage and disease progression. For an age-old disease that continues to afflict millions across the globe, new and effective treatments are certainly welcome. Moving from bench to bedside, and also switching from life sciences to biomedical technology, the third chapter on Respiratory Surface Electromyography (EMG) introduces translational research in pulmonary emphysema. EMG, hitherto more often within the purview of neurophysiology, may in the future play a significant role in clinical pulmonology as a noninvasive and comprehensive means of evaluating dyspnoea and respiratory effort—both essential parameters that are currently not easily measurable in clinical practice. The fourth chapter summarizes the general role of bronchoscopy, with special emphasis on safety and therapy in patients with emphysema. Next, a dissertation on lung deposition follows, discussing the significance of, factors affecting, and currently available methods of evaluation. Interestingly, the authors successfully synthesize their discussion on lung deposition of seemingly disparate but related themes in emphysema—air pollutants and inhaled medication—and even include a section on inhaled drug delivery in patients on noninvasive ventilation. The final chapter closes this textbook with a summary of lung transplantation for advanced (end-stage) lung disease. In this volume, the authors provide an excellent overview, while highlighting their exposition with aspects of lung transplantation pertaining to patients with COPD. To a nontransplant clinician, this review chapter is a longed-for erudition. In sum, I would like to acknowledge all of my expert collaborators' invaluable contributions to this textbook and also extend an appreciation to Valentina Jolić for overseeing the publishing process.

Kian Chung Ong
Chestmed Private Limited,
Mount Elizabeth Medical Centre,
Singapore

Chapter 1

Introductory Chapter: Contemporizing Chronic Obstructive Pulmonary Disease

Kian Chung Ong and Earnest Arul

1. Introduction

One characteristic of modernity is the belief that the more recent something is, the better and truer it must be. Chronocentrism, the assumption that the current time-period represents the best epoch throughout history, pervades societies of any age, but perhaps, such conceit affects this generation more than previous ones. With the onset of the Information Age, when new data can be proclaimed and widely assessed almost instantly, the hubris of living in the Golden Age of knowledge transfer and consensus creation is considerable. Nonetheless, readers of honorable vintage will recall certain promising discoveries in the past that did not stand the test of time, and likewise, established opinions that did not end up 'on the right side of history.' A medical condition with such a long history as Chronic Obstructive Pulmonary Disease (COPD) is expectedly fraught with controversies and swings in paradigms. The age-old tussle between an overlap or a continuum of asthma and COPD, and the recent publication followed by dissolution of global guidelines in managing asthma-COPD overlap are some examples of vagaries in current considerations of airway disorders. Of more contemporary interest are the recently proposed and adopted changes to the definition and taxonomy (classification) of COPD itself [1]. This chapter summarizes the recent revisions in the definition, terminology and taxonomy of COPD and proposes a theoretical viewpoint to make sense of contemporizing changes made to the essential notions of this ancient disease.

2. The transforming nosology of COPD and pulmonary emphysema

The terms "emphysema" or "pulmonary emphysema" predated COPD by decades. Bonet's description of "voluminous lungs" was written in 1679 [2]. In 1821, Laënnec, a clinician, pathologist and the inventor of the stethoscope, first designated the term "emphysema" to the findings of lungs that remained hyperinflated and did not empty well at autopsy. The first comprehensive textbook of pulmonary emphysema was published in 1956. During the period 1959–1962, the components of COPD – chronic bronchitis, emphysema and asthma were defined by colloquium. Over the intervening years till present, the clinical definition of COPD has been refined as emphysema continues to retain its description in anatomic terms.

The Global Strategy for Prevention, Diagnosis and Management of COPD, first issued about a quarter of a century ago, has recently revised its definition of

COPD [3]. In its latest iteration, COPD is defined as "a heterogeneous lung condition characterized by chronic respiratory symptoms (dyspnea, cough, expectoration) due to persistent abnormalities of the air ways (bronchitis, bronchiolitis), and/or alveoli (emphysema), that cause persistent, often progressive airflow obstruction". This new statement no longer requires the presence of demonstrable airflow limitation for defining COPD nor limits its causation to inhalation of noxious agents, viz., cigarette smoking. In addition, newer 'classes' of COPD reflecting underlying causes ("etiotypes") are included in a new taxonomy. These "etiotypes" are: genetically determined COPD, COPD due to abnormal lung development, environmental COPD, COPD caused by infections, COPD and asthma, and idiopathic COPD. In particular, the recently revised Global Strategy also emphasizes that COPD results from gene (G)- environment (E) interactions that occur over the lifetime (T) of an individual (ingeniously termed "GETomics"). The prime motivation behind these changes is the reduction of the obdurate morbidity and mortality in COPD, a process thought to be currently vitiated by delayed diagnosis resulting from a parochial definition and limited consideration accorded to pathogenetic factors. The effort to transform the basic tenets of COPD for the improvement of outcomes is laudable, as latest estimates of COPD disease burden (both current and future) are deplorable [4], especially when viewed against progress made for other major non-communicable diseases.

The most contentious among the recent revisions is the introduction of the following new terms – early COPD, mild COPD, young COPD, pre-COPD. These may lead to confusion rather than clarification, even though not all these newly defined entities are encouraged for use in clinical parlance, but in research settings only. Another novel term PRISm (preserved ratio impaired spirometry) describes findings of preserved FEV1/FVC ratio ≥ 0.7 but impaired spirometry (FEV1 $<$ 80% predicted), both indices after bronchodilation, is more likely to be utilized as it is a distinct and objectively defined entity.

It is noteworthy that, together with the revision in definition of COPD, the decades-long necessity for spirometry in the diagnosis of COPD has been removed from the new global guidelines [3]. In other words, spirometry is now desirable, but no longer "required" for diagnosing COPD, much like the case for bronchial asthma. This is in line with the goal to include disease in its early stages, before airflow obstruction is evident. However, the trade-offs for such inclusivity are the uncertainty of COPD diagnosis and the mislabeling of cases. Regarding these concerns, the researchers advising these recent revisions had argued that a nosologic entity such as COPD defined only in clinical-descriptive terms is valid, "provided that verbal usages are made explicit and applied consistently" [1]. It remains to be seen how well patients take to being diagnosed with COPD and classified accordingly in their "earlier" stages *without* any objective operational criteria.

Gratefully, amidst the recent wide-ranging nosologic changes, the term COPD is retained. The acronym COPD has taken decades for widespread acceptance among stake-holders and the wider public. COPD is now recognized by major global health organizations, widely used in the medical literature, and accepted in the Internal Coding of Diseases. Based on Google Trends, 'COPD' is an increasingly popular search term since the year 2004, especially compared to 'emphysema' (see **Figure 1**). The rising awareness and usage of the term COPD may presumably be credited to the foregoing annually-revised Global Strategy on COPD and other efforts by the Global Initiative for Chronic Obstructive Lung Disease (GOLD), which was established in 1999. Common sense has prevailed in maintaining this medical term (although not a most precise one) for which some educators have spent the length of a career in health communication.

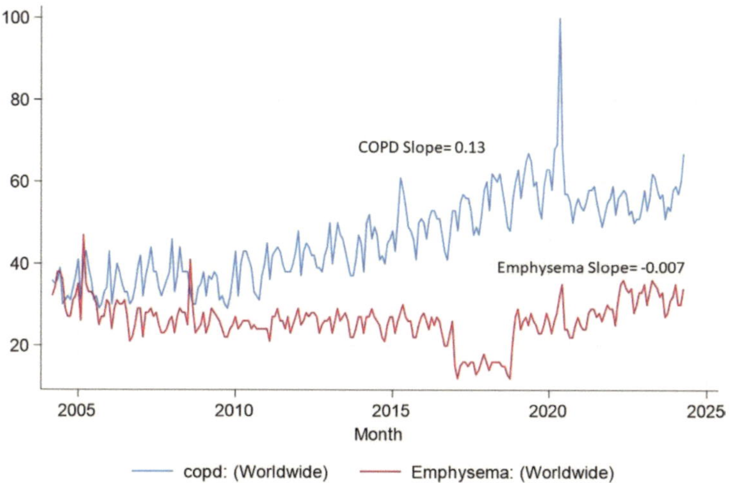

Figure 1.
Time plot using Google Trends showing frequency of search terms over time since 2004.

3. The prejudice of the universal

The recent revisions to the definition and nomenclature of COPD may be compared to another common predilection of modernity - a dichotomy between the universal and the particular. Moderns have been conditioned to value the universal and the abstract over the situated and the specific. This prejudice of the universal over the particular is expressed in the need for an all-encompassing definition of a condition as common and as heterogeneous as COPD. Yet, the more inclusive and general a definition has become, the greater the need for classification and sub-typing according to etiology and time of presentation, as we are presently witnessing. The complexity involved in diagnosing and treating a widespread and varied malady such as COPD requires contextualization as concepts of COPD vary according to global/local and synchronic/diachronic factors as previously described [5]. Recognizing the prejudice of the universal, it behooves clinicians to desist the devaluing of specific patient differences, even if it is deemed 'scandalous' to emphasize such differences beyond general characteristics of the disease.

4. Conclusion

The recent amendments to the definition and nomenclature of COPD represent broad changes to global guidelines that have been established for many years. These changes to the basic concepts and requirements in the diagnosis of COPD have major implications in research and clinical practice. Only time will tell if these revisions correspond to the unexamined modern notion of "the newer, the better".

Conflict of interest

The authors declare no conflict of interest.

Author details

Kian Chung Ong[1*] and Earnest Arul[2]

1 Chestmed Private Limited, Mount Elizabeth Medical Centre, Singapore

2 School of Public Health and Preventive Medicine, Monash University, Melbourne, VIC, Australia

*Address all correspondence to: ongkc@chestmed.com.sg

References

[1] Celli B, Fabbri L, Criner G, et al. Definition and nomenclature of chronic obstructive pulmonary disease: Time for its revision. American Journal of Respiratory and Critical Care Medicine. 2022;**206**(11):1317-1325. DOI: 10.1164/rccm.202204-0671PP

[2] Petty TL. The history of COPD. International Journal of Chronic Obstructive Pulmonary Disease. 2006;**1**(1):3-14. DOI: 10.2147/copd.2006.1.1.3

[3] Agustí A, Celli BR, Criner GJ, et al. Global initiative for chronic obstructive lung disease 2023 report: GOLD executive summary. American Journal of Respiratory and Critical Care Medicine. 2023;**207**(7):819-837. DOI: 10.1164/rccm.202301-0106PP

[4] Boers E, Barrett M, Su JG, et al. Global burden of chronic obstructive pulmonary disease through 2050. JAMA Network Open. 2023;**6**(12):e2346598. DOI: 10.1001/jamanetworkopen.2023.46598

[5] Ong KC. Introductory chapter: Contextualizing chronic obstructive pulmonary disease. In: A Compendium of Chronic Obstructive Pulmonary Disease. London, UK: IntechOpen; 2023. DOI: 10.5772/intechopen.109561

Chapter 2

The Intricate Involvement of Macrophages in Pulmonary Emphysema: Insights, Mechanisms, and Therapeutic Perspectives

Balachandar Selvakumar

Abstract

The intricate involvement of macrophages in pulmonary emphysema signifies their pivotal role in disease pathogenesis and progression. Dysregulated macrophage behavior, marked by altered activation states, promotes chronic inflammation, protease release, and oxidative stress, exacerbating tissue damage and alveolar destruction. Targeting macrophages emerges as a promising therapeutic avenue to modulate immune responses, restore tissue homeostasis, and mitigate disease severity. Recent advances have highlighted macrophage heterogeneity, signaling pathways, and their impact on lung tissue remodeling. Understanding the complexities of macrophage involvement offers insights into novel therapeutic strategies and potential interventions aimed at modulating their behavior to halt disease progression. Future prospects involve precision therapies, multi-target approaches, and comprehensive studies to validate the efficacy and safety of macrophage-targeted interventions, paving the way for transformative management strategies in pulmonary emphysema.

Keywords: macrophages, pulmonary emphysema, inflammation, therapeutic targets, disease progression

1. Introduction

Chronic obstructive pulmonary disease (COPD) is a multifaceted respiratory disorder characterized by irreversible airflow limitation, where pulmonary emphysema stands as a significant pathological feature [1, 2]. Macrophages emerge as pivotal players within this complex intricate disease landscape, orchestrating a delicate balance between lung homeostasis and destructive inflammation [3]. This chapter delves into the profound interplay between macrophages and pulmonary emphysema, unraveling their nuanced roles, underlying mechanisms, and the promising therapeutic avenues they unveil. From their foundational functions in healthy lung physiology to their dysregulated behavior in the diseased state, the involvement of macrophages holds both the keys to understanding disease progression and the promise of targeted interventions. Exploration of macrophage phenotypes, their intricate interaction networks, and their impact on lung tissue integrity unveils the complex dynamics driving emphysematous changes. From their pivotal role in immune responses to their contribution to proteolytic cascades and oxidative stress, the multifaceted nature of macrophages in driving tissue damage becomes apparent. In light of this complex interplay, this chapter navigates through emerging research, therapeutic strategies, and the challenges posed in targeting macrophages for therapeutic benefit. By scrutinizing experimental models, recent breakthroughs, and potential interventions, this exploration seeks to shed light on novel avenues for combating the relentless progression of pulmonary emphysema. Amidst the complexities lie opportunities, and herein lies the exploration of macrophage involvement in pulmonary emphysema—a journey encompassing insights, mechanisms, and the promising vistas of therapeutic perspectives.

1.1 Overview of pulmonary emphysema

Pulmonary emphysema represents a debilitating condition within the spectrum of COPD, characterized by irreversible damage to the lung's air sacs (alveoli) and progressive impairment of respiratory function [4]. This disease manifests through the destruction of alveolar walls, leading to enlarged airspaces, decreased elasticity of lung tissue, and compromised gas exchange. Emphysema typically results from prolonged exposure to noxious particles or gases, notably cigarette smoke, causing chronic inflammation and oxidative stress in the lungs [5]. Clinically, patients experience dyspnea, coughing, and reduced exercise tolerance as the disease advances. Emphysema significantly impacts respiratory mechanics, impairing the expulsion of air from the lungs and causing hyperinflation [6]. Understanding the pathological alterations in lung structure and function characteristic of pulmonary emphysema is crucial for devising targeted interventions and therapeutic strategies aimed at managing this debilitating respiratory condition.

1.2 Importance of macrophages in lung physiology and pathology

Macrophages hold a pivotal role in maintaining lung homeostasis, contributing significantly to both physiological functions and pathological responses within the pulmonary microenvironment [3]. In lung physiology, these versatile immune cells serve as key sentinels, patrolling the airways and alveoli to clear inhaled particles, pathogens, and cellular debris. Beyond their role in host defense, macrophages actively participate in tissue repair, contributing to the clearance of apoptotic cells and promoting resolution of inflammation [7]. Their capacity to modulate immune responses, release signaling molecules, and regulate tissue remodeling underscores their importance in orchestrating a delicate balance between immune surveillance and tolerance within the lungs. However, in the context of lung pathology such as pulmonary emphysema, macrophages exhibit dysregulated behaviors. Prolonged exposure to harmful agents, such as cigarette smoke or environmental pollutants, can lead to an altered macrophage phenotype, marked by increased pro-inflammatory responses, impaired phagocytic function, and the release of destructive enzymes and reactive oxygen species. This dysregulated macrophage behavior contributes significantly to the progression of lung diseases, amplifying inflammation and tissue damage and exacerbating respiratory dysfunction [8]. Understanding the dichotomous roles of macrophages in lung physiology and pathology is crucial for unraveling their contributions to disease progression and identifying therapeutic avenues to restore immune balance and mitigate tissue damage in lung disorders.

1.3 Objective and scope of the chapter

The primary objective of this chapter is to comprehensively explore and elucidate the intricate involvement of macrophages in the pathogenesis, progression, and potential therapeutic interventions in pulmonary emphysema. By delving into the multifaceted roles of macrophages within the pulmonary microenvironment, this chapter aims to dissect their contributions to disease mechanisms, including inflammation, tissue destruction, and immune dysregulation. Moreover, the chapter seeks to underscore the impact of macrophage dysfunction on disease severity, offering insights into potential targets for therapeutic modulation and interventions aimed at restoring immune homeostasis and mitigating lung tissue damage in pulmonary emphysema.

This chapter will delineate the diversity of macrophage phenotypes present in pulmonary emphysema, exploring their functional diversity, plasticity, and the intricacies of their roles in maintaining lung homeostasis and contributing to disease pathology. In addition, it will elucidate the underlying mechanisms through which macrophages exacerbate tissue destruction, including the release of proteases, oxidative stress, and their interactions with other immune cells and structural components of the lung. The chapter will analyze the impact of macrophage-driven inflammation and immune dysregulation on disease progression, emphasizing their role in perpetuating chronic inflammation and impairing tissue repair mechanisms. Moreover, it will discuss current and emerging therapeutic strategies aimed at modulating macrophage behavior, restoring immune balance, and mitigating lung tissue damage. This includes pharmacological interventions, potential drug targets, and innovative approaches for targeting macrophages in the treatment of pulmonary emphysema. Finally, the chapter will address challenges in targeting macrophages therapeutically, potential limitations, and future research directions required to further elucidate the complexities of macrophage involvement and develop effective therapeutic interventions for pulmonary emphysema.

2. Pathogenesis of pulmonary emphysema

The pathogenesis of pulmonary emphysema is multifactorial, involving intricate interactions between environmental exposures, inflammatory responses, and structural alterations in lung tissue.

2.1 Etiology and risk factors

Pulmonary emphysema is primarily associated with prolonged exposure to noxious particles or gases, notably cigarette smoke, which remains the leading cause worldwide [9]. Other risk factors include occupational exposures to pollutants, genetic predispositions, and alpha-1 antitrypsin deficiency. These factors lead to chronic inflammation and oxidative stress within the lungs, triggering a cascade of events that result in alveolar destruction and impaired repair mechanisms [9].

2.2 Structural changes in the lung parenchyma

The hallmark of pulmonary emphysema is the irreversible destruction of the alveolar walls, leading to enlarged airspaces and decreased elasticity of lung tissue. This pathological process involves the breakdown of the alveolar septa, which normally provide structural support and maintain the alveolar structure [10]. The loss of these walls results in the coalescence of small airspaces into larger ones, diminishing the lung's surface area for gas exchange and impairing its elastic recoil.

2.3 Role of inflammation and immune responses

Chronic inflammation plays a pivotal role in emphysema pathogenesis. In response to noxious stimuli, resident immune cells, including macrophages, neutrophils, and T lymphocytes, are activated, leading to the release of pro-inflammatory cytokines and proteolytic enzymes [11–13]. These inflammatory mediators perpetuate tissue damage by activating pathways that degrade the extracellular matrix, particularly elastin, essential for maintaining lung elasticity. Moreover, oxidative stress induced by the production of reactive oxygen species further exacerbates tissue injury and impairs repair mechanisms, contributing to the perpetuation of alveolar destruction [14].

Overall, the pathogenesis of pulmonary emphysema involves a complex interplay between environmental insults, inflammatory responses, and structural alterations in lung tissue. Understanding these intricate mechanisms is critical for developing targeted interventions aimed at mitigating inflammation, preserving lung architecture, and restoring lung function in individuals affected by this debilitating respiratory condition.

3. Macrophage biology in lung homeostasis

Macrophages play pivotal roles in maintaining tissue homeostasis, contributing to immune surveillance, tissue repair, and modulation of inflammatory responses [7]. Their functional diversity, phenotypic plasticity, and activation states underscore their significance in lung physiology.

3.1 Functions of tissue macrophages

Macrophages patrol the airways and alveoli, clearing inhaled particles, pathogens, and cellular debris, acting as the first line of defense against respiratory threats. Macrophages regulate immune responses by secreting cytokines, chemokines, and growth factors, influencing the activation and function of other immune cells within the lung microenvironment. These cells can facilitate tissue repair by phagocytosing apoptotic cells, assisting in extracellular matrix turnover, and promoting resolution of inflammation to restore lung architecture after injury by releasing various pro-repair mediators and growth factors [7].

3.2 Plasticity of macrophages

Macrophages demonstrate remarkable plasticity, transitioning between activation states in response to microenvironmental cues. This plasticity enables them to adapt their functional phenotypes, allowing for a dynamic response to changing microenvironmental signals [15]. Macrophages exhibit phenotypic diversity influenced by their microenvironment, displaying a spectrum of activation states ranging from classical (M1) to alternative (M2) activation, each associated with distinct functional profiles [16]. Inflammatory stimuli like lipopolysaccharide (LPS) or interferon-gamma (IFN-γ) induce M1 phenotype and secrete pro-inflammatory cytokines like TNF-α, IL-1β, and IL-6, promoting microbicidal activity. Macrophages that are exposed to anti-inflammatory signals such as IL-4 or IL-13 drive themselves to M2 phenotype and exhibit tissue repair, immunoregulatory, and anti-inflammatory functions. They release cytokines like IL-10 and TGF-β, contributing to tissue healing and suppressing inflammation. However, an unbalanced secretion of these anti- and pro-inflammatory mediators could cause tissue destructive- and remodeling-associated disease conditions.

Understanding the intricacies of macrophage biology in lung homeostasis, including their diverse functions, phenotypic plasticity, and activation states, is pivotal for comprehending their contributions to lung diseases like pulmonary emphysema. Dysregulated macrophage behavior can significantly impact disease pathogenesis, highlighting the importance of modulating their responses for therapeutic interventions in lung disorders.

4. Mechanisms of macrophage-mediated lung damage

Macrophages, crucial components of the lung's immune defense, wield a paradoxical influence on tissue integrity. While essential for pathogen clearance and tissue repair, dysregulated or chronically activated macrophages can induce substantial damage to lung tissue. Their uncontrolled activation causes the release of inflammatory molecules, such as cytokines and reactive species and can incite a cascade of events leading to inflammation, extracellular matrix degradation, and compromised structural integrity. These cells, when interacting with neutrophils or epithelial cells, can exacerbate tissue injury through amplified inflammatory responses and impaired repair mechanisms. Consequently, in chronic conditions like COPD or certain infections, macrophages play a pivotal role in precipitating alveolar destruction and airspace enlargement, ultimately contributing to the pathogenesis of respiratory diseases characterized by tissue degradation.

4.1 Altered macrophage phenotype in emphysematous lungs

In emphysematous lungs, the phenotype and behavior of macrophages undergo profound alterations, contributing significantly to disease progression. Prolonged exposure to noxious agents, such as cigarette smoke, induces a shift in macrophage activation, leading to a dysregulated phenotype characterized by an imbalance between pro-inflammatory and reparative functions [8, 9]. These altered macrophages, often skewed toward an M1-like pro-inflammatory state, display impaired phagocytic activity, reduced capacity for resolving inflammation, and an augmented release of proteases and reactive oxygen species. For example, an excess secretion of MMP-12 (macrophage elastase) by alveolar macrophages is known to mediate the development of lung injury and emphysema [17].

This skewed activation state perpetuates chronic inflammation, exacerbates tissue damage, and compromises repair mechanisms, fostering an environment conducive to alveolar destruction and impaired lung function. Understanding and targeting these altered macrophage phenotypes in emphysema are critical for developing therapeutic strategies aimed at modulating their behavior, restoring immune balance, and mitigating lung tissue damage in this debilitating respiratory condition.

4.2 Impaired phagocytic activity and clearance of cellular debris

In pulmonary emphysema, impaired phagocytic activity and compromised clearance of cellular debris by macrophages significantly contribute to disease pathology. Macrophages, critical in maintaining lung homeostasis, typically phagocytose cellular remnants, debris, and apoptotic cells, play a pivotal role in tissue repair and resolution of inflammation. However, in emphysematous lungs, this essential function is hindered [17].

Prolonged exposure to noxious stimuli, especially cigarette smoke, leads to alterations in macrophage phenotypes, reducing their ability to efficiently clear apoptotic cells and debris. Dysfunctional macrophages in emphysema exhibit diminished expression of phagocytic receptors and impaired recognition of apoptotic cells [18]. Consequently, the clearance of cellular debris becomes compromised, allowing the accumulation of apoptotic cells, extracellular matrix fragments, and other debris within the lung microenvironment. This impaired phagocytic activity not only disrupts tissue repair mechanisms but also perpetuates inflammation. The accumulation of apoptotic cells and debris triggers an inflammatory response, perpetuating a cycle of tissue damage and chronic inflammation, exacerbating the progression of emphysematous changes in the lung parenchyma [19].

Restoring efficient phagocytic function in macrophages represents a potential therapeutic target in pulmonary emphysema. Strategies aimed at enhancing macrophage phagocytosis and clearance mechanisms could mitigate tissue damage, resolve inflammation, and potentially halt the progression of this debilitating respiratory condition.

4.3 Inflammatory responses and release of protease

In pulmonary emphysema, macrophages play a pivotal role in perpetuating inflammation through intricate signaling pathways and exacerbate tissue damage *via* oxidative stress and the generation of reactive oxygen species (ROS) [20, 21]. Activated macrophages in emphysematous lungs stimulate inflammatory signaling cascades, including nuclear factor-kappa B (NF-κB) and mitogen-activated protein kinase (MAPK) pathways [22, 23]. These pathways drive the production and release of pro-inflammatory cytokines such as tumor necrosis factor-alpha (TNF-α), interleukin-1 beta (IL-1β), and interleukin-6 (IL-6), amplifying the inflammatory milieu within the lung microenvironment [20]. Moreover, macrophage-derived ROS, including superoxide anion and hydrogen peroxide, contribute to oxidative stress. The excessive production of ROS overwhelms antioxidant defenses, inducing cellular damage, lipid peroxidation, and DNA alterations [24]. This oxidative stress exacerbates inflammation, disrupts cellular functions, and contributes significantly to lung tissue injury, fostering the progressive destruction of alveolar structures characteristic of pulmonary emphysema. In pulmonary emphysema, macrophages produce an array of pro-inflammatory cytokines (such as TNF-α, IL-1β, IL-6, iNOS, COX-2, and chemokines (like CXCL8)) in emphysematous lungs. These molecules recruit and activate other immune cells, perpetuating the inflammatory cascade and contributing to tissue damage [20]. In addition, macrophages generate ROS as part of their inflammatory response. Excessive ROS production contributes to oxidative stress, causing damage to cellular components and exacerbating tissue injury [20, 21].

Macrophages contribute significantly to the inflammatory milieu through the release of various proteases, exacerbating tissue damage and perpetuating the progression of the disease. The altered phenotype of macrophages in emphysematous lungs, influenced by chronic exposure to noxious agents like cigarette smoke, leads to dysregulated immune responses, notably an increase in pro-inflammatory mediators and proteases. Macrophages in emphysematous lungs release elevated levels of matrix metalloproteinases (MMPs), particularly MMP-2, MMP-9, and MMP-12 [25]. These proteases target the extracellular matrix components, including elastin, collagen, and proteoglycans, contributing to the breakdown of alveolar walls and impairing lung tissue integrity [26]. In addition, macrophages release neutrophil elastase, further amplifying the proteolytic cascade. Neutrophil elastase cleaves elastin fibers [27], leading to loss of lung elasticity and airspace enlargement, characteristic of emphysema.

The sustained release of proteases and inflammatory mediators by macrophages in emphysema results in an imbalance between tissue destruction and repair mechanisms. This chronic inflammatory state perpetuates alveolar destruction, impairs tissue healing, and disrupts the delicate lung architecture, ultimately leading to the characteristic airspace enlargement seen in pulmonary emphysema. Targeting the dysregulated release of proteases and inflammatory mediators from macrophages represents a potential therapeutic strategy to mitigate tissue damage and halt disease progression in pulmonary emphysema. Understanding and targeting these pathways involved in macrophage-driven inflammation and oxidative stress may offer potential therapeutic avenues for mitigating tissue damage and managing the progression of emphysematous changes in the lungs.

4.4 Interaction with other cells

In emphysema, macrophages become activated due to exposure to irritants like cigarette smoke, pollution, or other inhaled toxins. These activated macrophages interact with various cell types in the lung microenvironment and influence lung tissue damage and promote the development of emphysematous lungs.

Neutrophils: Macrophages can interact with neutrophils to regulate inflammation and tissue repair. In response to tissue damage and inflammation, neutrophils are recruited to the lungs. Macrophages and neutrophils often collaborate in immune responses. However, dysregulated interactions between these cells may lead to increased inflammation and tissue injury due to excessive release of inflammatory molecules and oxidative stress. For example, abnormal apoptotic events in smokers' and in emphysematous lungs by macrophages are observed to contribute to the development of emphysema [28].

Epithelial Cells: Macrophages interact with epithelial cells through cytokines, chemokines, and cell–cell contacts. Dysfunctional crosstalk between macrophages and epithelial cells can contribute to tissue damage and impaired repair mechanisms [28].

Macrophages can influence fibroblast activity, affecting the repair processes in emphysematous lungs. T cells also interact with macrophages, modulating the inflammation in emphysema (**Figure 1**).

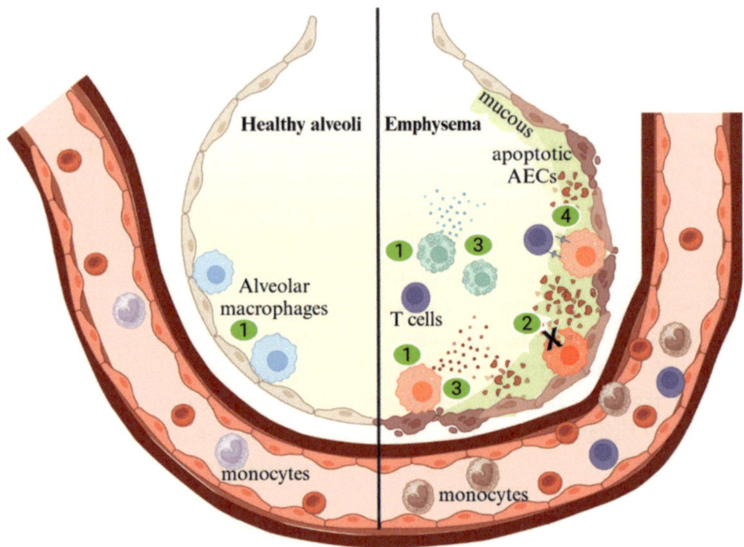

Figure 1.
Mechanisms of macrophage-mediated lung damage. Schematic diagram shows the healthy alveoli in the left side with resident alveolar macrophages maintaining alveolar homeostasis. The right side of the diagram shows the emphysema alveoli with enlarged alveolar space due to series of tissue damage majorly mediated by macrophages such as (1) altered phenotypes, (2) reduced or inhibited phagocytic activity, (3) release of pro-inflammatory cytokines and tissue destructive proteases, and (4) interaction with other cell types within the alveoli resulting in tissue destruction.

5. Targeting macrophages as therapeutic strategy

Targeting macrophages has emerged as a potential therapeutic strategy for treating emphysema. Since macrophages play a crucial role in the inflammatory response and tissue damage seen in emphysema, several approaches are being explored to modulate their function for therapeutic benefit.

5.1 Modulation of macrophage polarization

Macrophages have different activation states, broadly classified as M1 (pro-inflammatory) and M2 (anti-inflammatory/reparative). Shifting the balance from M1 to M2 phenotype can potentially reduce inflammation and promote tissue repair. This could be achieved through pharmacological agents or biological factors to promote a reparative response, fostering tissue repair and reducing inflammation [29]. In an *in vivo* study, a nature product propolis was observed to reverse the cigarette smoke-induced emphysema through macrophage alternative activation [30]. However, currently, there are very few studies available and there is huge demand in this area of research.

5.2 Phagocytic enhancement

Enhancing macrophage phagocytosis and clearance of apoptotic cells and debris is being investigated [31]. Stimulating phagocytic receptors or using nanoparticles to enhance debris clearance might mitigate tissue damage [32]. However, these studies have to be tightly regulated to prevent the exaggerated phagocytosis that can increase the severity of the disease.

5.3 Anti-inflammatory agents

Drugs that specifically target inflammatory pathways in macrophages can help reduce their activation and the subsequent release of inflammatory mediators. This approach aims to dampen the chronic inflammation seen in emphysema. Corticosteroids and inhibitors targeting specific inflammatory pathways, such as TNF-α or IL-1β antagonists, are under scrutiny to dampen excessive inflammation and limit tissue damage [33, 34]. Moreover, compounds with antioxidant properties, like N-acetylcysteine (NAC) or natural antioxidants, are explored to counteract oxidative stress and reduce ROS-mediated tissue injury [35, 36].

Moreover, macrophages release proteases that contribute to tissue destruction in emphysema. Inhibiting these proteases may help preserve lung structure and function [37]. However further studies are demanding. In addition, growing evidence has shown promising results with stem cell therapies. Therefore, exploring the use of stem cells to modulate macrophage activity and promote tissue repair in emphysema can add further advancement in the treatment strategies. Recent studies have showed that mesenchymal stem cells (MSCs) or their extracellular vesicles are observed to interact with macrophages and skew them to a tissue repair phenotype to resolve inflammation and induce repair mechanisms [38–40].

Clinical trials are underway to test the efficacy and safety of various drugs and interventions targeting macrophages in emphysema. However, the complexity of the disease and the multifaceted role of macrophages require a thorough understanding of their behavior in the context of emphysema to develop effective targeted therapies.

6. Emerging therapies and future directions

Recent advances in understanding macrophage dynamics in emphysema taking advantages of advanced techniques like single-cell RNA sequencing, researchers have identified distinct macrophage subpopulations in emphysematous lungs, delineating their heterogeneity, activation states, and functional diversity. In addition, imaging technologies with high-resolution imaging methods, such as intravital microscopy and multiphoton microscopy, enable real-time visualization of macrophage behavior in the lung microenvironment, offering insights into their interactions and responses during disease progression. Furthermore, metabolic profiling studies focusing on the metabolic reprogramming of macrophages in emphysema highlight alterations in their metabolic pathways, unveiling potential therapeutic targets to modulate macrophage function. These research advances in experimental models and technological innovations offer a deeper understanding of macrophage dynamics in pulmonary emphysema. By elucidating the complexities of macrophage responses and their impact on disease progression, these insights pave the way for the development of targeted therapies aimed at modulating macrophage behavior and managing emphysematous lung disease.

Biological therapies using monoclonal antibodies targeting specific macrophage receptors like IL-5, IL-7, PD-1, IL-19 [41–44], or signaling pathways [45, 46] are under investigation to modulate macrophage behavior and immune responses selectively. In addition, cell-based therapies utilizing stem cells or engineered macrophages to promote tissue repair, modulate inflammation, or enhance phagocytic activity show promise as an innovative therapeutic approach [39, 40].

In addition, the role of the microbiota in influencing macrophages in emphysema and COPD is an area of growing research interest. The respiratory tract is not sterile, and the lung microbiota can modulate the immune response and contribute to the pathogenesis of lung diseases, including emphysema and COPD. Studies suggest that alterations in the lung microbiota composition may contribute to inflammation in COPD and emphysema [47]. Changes in microbial diversity and abundance may influence the activation state of macrophages. The lung microbiota can influence macrophage function by interacting with pattern recognition receptors (PRRs) on macrophages. PRRs recognize microbial components, leading to the activation of macrophages and the release of inflammatory mediators [7]. Moreover, microbial metabolites produced by the lung microbiota can have immunomodulatory effects. Short-chain fatty acids (SCFAs), for example, are microbial metabolites that have been shown to influence macrophage polarization and function. Dysbiosis, an imbalance in the composition of the microbiota, has been associated with COPD and emphysema [48]. Dysbiosis may contribute to chronic inflammation and alter the local immune response, including the activity of macrophages.

In the future, modulating the lung microbiota has been proposed as a therapeutic strategy for COPD and emphysema. Probiotics, prebiotics, and fecal microbiota transplantation are being explored to restore microbial balance and potentially influence macrophage behavior. Tailoring therapies based on individual disease phenotypes and patient-specific characteristics might enhance treatment efficacy and add advances in precision medicine. Moreover, multi-target approaches including combining therapies targeting different aspects of macrophage dysfunction, inflammation, and tissue repair pathways could offer synergistic benefits in managing pulmonary emphysema. In parallel, comprehensive long-term studies focusing on safety, efficacy, and the potential for disease modification are needed to validate the therapeutic strategies targeting macrophages in pulmonary emphysema. Harnessing these therapeutic strategies targeting macrophages, inflammatory pathways, and oxidative stress holds promise in altering disease progression, preserving lung function, and ameliorating the burden of pulmonary emphysema. However, further research and clinical trials are essential to validate their efficacy, safety, and long-term impact in managing this complex respiratory condition.

7. Experimental models

Experimental models play a crucial role in understanding macrophage involvement and dynamics in pulmonary emphysema (**Table 1**). Several animal models have been utilized to study the role of macrophages. (1) Smoke-induced models in which exposure of rodents (mice or rats) to cigarette smoke (CS), mimicking the chronic exposure seen in human smokers. These models replicate emphysematous changes, including airspace enlargement, inflammation, and altered macrophage phenotypes, resembling human emphysema pathophysiology [57]. These models provide better mimicking features with human emphysema; nevertheless, the duration of the models require a long period exposure, (2) enzyme-induced models, where intratracheal administration of proteolytic enzymes like elastase or papain induces alveolar damage and emphysematous changes, allowing for the study of macrophage responses and disease progression [49, 50]. These models can provide simple methodology with low cost; however, the consistency with human emphysema is not satisfactory, and (3) Genetically modified models, which usually use transgenic or gene knockout

Induction substance	Mode of administration	Animal	Mechanism	References
Elastase (papain, pig pancreatic elastinase (PPE), and human neutrophil elastase (HNE)	Intratracheal	Tat and hamster	Elastase disrupts protease–antiprotease balance and accelerates the rupture and fusion of alveolar walls to induce emphysema.	[49, 50]
Passive smoking	Smoke stimulation (part exposure: nose or head only)	Guinea pig, C57BL/6J mice	Long-term CS exposure induces inflammatory responses leading to narrowing of bronchial lumen and cartilage tissue, causing rupture and fusion of alveoli and the formation of emphysema, mimicking human conditions	[51, 52]
Chemicals (NO_2, lipopolysaccharides (LPS), O_3, and cadmium chloride ($CdCl_2$), of hyaluronidase, ovalbumin dry powder)	Inhalation, intratracheal, and intravenous injection.	C57BL/6 mice, Wistar rats, Guinea pigs, golden ground squirrels	NO2, common in air pollution, induces emphysema by the overproduction of oxidative stress. Mechanisms of other agents are unknown	[53–56]
Cigarette smoke extract	Intraperitoneal injection	Mice and rats	Intraperitoneal injection of CSE increases alveolar space, alveolar wall destruction, apoptosis of alveolar septum cells, and chronic lung inflammation and promotes pulmonary dysfunction.	[57]
Genetic manipulation (Platelet-derived growth factor-β (PDGF-β), TNF-α, IL-6, and IL-11	Gene-targeted and/or genetically modified	Usually mice	Loss or hindered function of these genes impairs the normal development of alveoli. Excessive expression of certain genes like PDGF-β may disrupt the balance between alveolar damage and repair, leading to emphysema.	[58, 59]

Table 1.
Animal models of emphysema.

technology by which targeting specific genes associated with macrophage function or inflammation aids in understanding the mechanistic aspects of macrophage involvement in emphysema development [58, 59]. Although these models can be more models can be targeted to understand function of genes, they demand high-end techniques with high costs.

8. Conclusion

Macrophages serve as central players in the pathogenesis of pulmonary emphysema, orchestrating a delicate balance between immune surveillance and tissue repair. Their dysregulated activation states and inflammatory responses profoundly impact disease progression, influencing the destruction and remodeling of lung parenchyma. Understanding their multifaceted roles offers insights into potential therapeutic interventions targeting macrophages to alleviate tissue damage and halt disease progression.

Macrophages in pulmonary emphysema exhibit altered phenotypes, skewed toward pro-inflammatory states, impairing phagocytosis and promoting release of proteases and oxidative stress. Their dysregulated behavior perpetuates chronic inflammation, exacerbating tissue damage, contributing significantly to alveolar destruction, and impairing repair mechanisms. Targeting macrophages emerges as a promising therapeutic strategy, aiming to modulate their behavior, restore immune balance, and mitigate tissue damage in emphysematous lungs.

Unraveling the intricate involvement of macrophages in pulmonary emphysema sheds light on novel avenues for therapeutic intervention. While significant strides have been made, there is a need for (1) tailoring interventions based on patient-specific phenotypes for improved efficacy in a Precision Therapy approach, (2) combination therapies targeting multiple aspects of macrophage dysfunction and tissue repair pathways, and (3) comprehensive investigations assessing safety, efficacy, and disease-modifying potential of macrophage-targeted therapies by long-term studies. Looking ahead, harnessing the potential of targeted macrophage modulation and innovative therapies and advancing our understanding of macrophage behavior holds promise in reshaping the management and outlook for individuals affected by pulmonary emphysema. This comprehensive understanding of macrophage involvement paves the way for transformative approaches aimed at attenuating disease progression and improving clinical outcomes in this challenging respiratory condition.

Author details

Balachandar Selvakumar
Research Institute of Medical and Health Sciences (RIMHS), College of Medicine, University of Sharjah, United Arab Emirates

*Address all correspondence to: bselvakumar@sharjah.ac.ae

References

[1] Guo P, Li R, Piao TH, Wang CL, Wu XL, Cai HY. Pathological mechanism and targeted drugs of COPD. International Journal of Chronic Obstructive Pulmonary Disease. 2022;**17**:1565-1575

[2] Hisata S, Racanelli AC, Kermani P, Schreiner R, Houghton S, Palikuqi B, et al. Reversal of emphysema by restoration of pulmonary endothelial cells. The Journal of Experimental Medicine. 2 Aug 2021;**218**(8):e20200938

[3] Malainou C, Abdin SM, Lachmann N, Matt U, Herold S. Alveolar macrophages in tissue homeostasis, inflammation, and infection: Evolving concepts of therapeutic targeting. The Journal of Clinical Investigation. 2 Oct 2023;**133**(19):e170501

[4] Bagdonas E, Raudoniute J, Bruzauskaite I, Aldonyte R. Novel aspects of pathogenesis and regeneration mechanisms in COPD. International Journal of Chronic Obstructive Pulmonary Disease. 2015;**10**:995-1013

[5] Hogg JC, Timens W. The pathology of chronic obstructive pulmonary disease. Annual Review of Pathology. 2009;**4**:435-459

[6] Cosio MG, Cosio Piqueras MG. Pathology of emphysema in chronic obstructive pulmonary disease. Monaldi Archives for Chest Disease. 2000;**55**(2):124-129

[7] Selvakumar B, Sekar P, Samsudin R. Intestinal macrophages in pathogenesis and treatment of gut leakage: Current strategies and future perspectives. Journal of Leukocyte Biology. 10 Jan 2024:qiad165

[8] Kapellos TS, Bassler K, Aschenbrenner AC, Fujii W, Schultze JL. Dysregulated functions of lung macrophage populations in COPD. Journal of Immunology Research. 2018;**2018**:2349045

[9] Demedts IK, Demoor T, Bracke KR, Joos GF, Brusselle GG. Role of apoptosis in the pathogenesis of COPD and pulmonary emphysema. Respiratory Research. 2006;**7**(1):53

[10] Benlala I, Laurent F, Dournes G. Structural and functional changes in COPD: What we have learned from imaging. Respirology. 2021;**26**(8):731-741

[11] Craig JM, Scott AL, Mitzner W. Immune-mediated inflammation in the pathogenesis of emphysema: Insights from mouse models. Cell and Tissue Research. 2017;**367**(3):591-605

[12] Lugg ST, Scott A, Parekh D, Naidu B, Thickett DR. Cigarette smoke exposure and alveolar macrophages: Mechanisms for lung disease. Thorax. 2022;**77**(1):94-101

[13] Kim YH, Choi YJ, Kang MK, Park SH, Antika LD, Lee EJ, et al. Astragalin inhibits allergic inflammation and airway thickening in ovalbumin-challenged mice. Journal of Agricultural and Food Chemistry. 2017;**65**(4):836-845

[14] Deslee G, Woods JC, Moore C, Conradi SH, Gierada DS, Atkinson JJ, et al. Oxidative damage to nucleic acids in severe emphysema. Chest. 2009;**135**(4):965-974

[15] Hussell T, Bell TJ. Alveolar macrophages: Plasticity in a tissue-specific context. Nature Reviews. Immunology. 2014;**14**(2):81-93

[16] Yunna C, Mengru H, Lei W, Weidong C. Macrophage M1/

M2 polarization. European Journal of Pharmacology. 2020;**877**:173090

[17] Spix B, Butz ES, Chen CC, Rosato AS, Tang R, Jeridi A, et al. Lung emphysema and impaired macrophage elastase clearance in mucolipin 3 deficient mice. Nature Communications. 2022;**13**(1):318

[18] Tanno A, Fujino N, Yamada M, Sugiura H, Hirano T, Tanaka R, et al. Decreased expression of a phagocytic receptor Siglec-1 on alveolar macrophages in chronic obstructive pulmonary disease. Respiratory Research. 2020;**21**(1):30

[19] Lee J, Lu Y, Oshins R, West J, Moneypenny CG, Han K, et al. Alpha 1 antitrypsin-deficient macrophages have impaired efferocytosis of apoptotic neutrophils. Frontiers in Immunology. 2020;**11**:574410

[20] Lee JW, Chun W, Lee HJ, Min JH, Kim SM, Seo JY, et al. The role of macrophages in the development of acute and chronic inflammatory lung diseases. Cell. 2021;**10**(4)

[21] Finicelli M, Digilio FA, Galderisi U, Peluso G. The emerging role of macrophages in chronic obstructive pulmonary disease: The potential impact of oxidative stress and extracellular vesicle on macrophage polarization and function. Antioxidants (Basel). 26 Feb 2022;**11**(3):464

[22] Renda T, Baraldo S, Pelaia G, Bazzan E, Turato G, Papi A, et al. Increased activation of p38 MAPK in COPD. The European Respiratory Journal. 2008;**31**(1):62-69

[23] Edwards MR, Bartlett NW, Clarke D, Birrell M, Belvisi M, Johnston SL. Targeting the NF-kappaB pathway in asthma and chronic obstructive pulmonary disease. Pharmacology & Therapeutics. 2009;**121**(1):1-13

[24] Forte A, Finicelli M, Grossi M, Vicchio M, Alessio N, Santé P, et al. DNA damage and repair in a model of rat vascular injury. Clinical Science (London, England). 2010;**118**(7):473-485

[25] Yoshida M, Whitsett JA. Alveolar macrophages and emphysema in surfactant protein-D-deficient mice. Respirology. 2006;**11**(Suppl):S37-S40

[26] Lu P, Takai K, Weaver VM, Werb Z. Extracellular matrix degradation and remodeling in development and disease. Cold Spring Harbor Perspectives in Biology. 1 Dec 2011;**3**(12):a005058

[27] McGowan SE, Stone PJ, Calore JD, Snider GL, Franzblau C. The fate of neutrophil elastase incorporated by human alveolar macrophages. The American Review of Respiratory Disease. 1983;**127**(4):449-455

[28] Plataki M, Tzortzaki E, Rytila P, Demosthenes M, Koutsopoulos A, Siafakas NM. Apoptotic mechanisms in the pathogenesis of COPD. International Journal of Chronic Obstructive Pulmonary Disease. 2006;**1**(2):161-171

[29] Feng H, Yin Y, Zheng R, Kang J. Rosiglitazone ameliorated airway inflammation induced by cigarette smoke via inhibiting the M1 macrophage polarization by activating PPARγ and RXRα. International Immunopharmacology. 2021;**97**:107809

[30] Barroso MV, Cattani-Cavalieri I, de Brito-Gitirana L, Fautrel A, Lagente V, Schmidt M, et al. Propolis reversed cigarette smoke-induced emphysema through macrophage alternative activation independent of Nrf2. Bioorganic & Medicinal Chemistry. 2017;**25**(20):5557-5568

[31] Chang CF, Massey J, Osherov A, Angenendt da Costa LH, Sansing LH. Bexarotene enhances macrophage erythrophagocytosis and hematoma clearance in experimental intracerebral hemorrhage. Stroke. 2020;**51**(2):612-618

[32] Ramesh A, Kumar S, Nguyen A, Brouillard A, Kulkarni A. Lipid-based phagocytosis nanoenhancer for macrophage immunotherapy. Nanoscale. 2020;**12**(3):1875-1885

[33] Lea S, Higham A, Beech A, Singh D. How inhaled corticosteroids target inflammation in COPD. European Respiratory Review. 18 Oct 2023;**32**(170):230084

[34] Kubo H, Asai K, Kojima K, Sugitani A, Kyomoto Y, Okamoto A, et al. Astaxanthin suppresses cigarette smoke-induced emphysema through Nrf2 activation in mice. Marine Drugs. 28 Nov 2019;**17**(12):673

[35] Xie C, Yi J, Lu J, Nie M, Huang M, Rong J, et al. N-acetylcysteine reduces ROS-mediated oxidative DNA damage and PI3K/Akt pathway activation induced by *Helicobacter pylori* infection. Oxidative Medicine and Cellular Longevity. 2018;**2018**:1874985

[36] Xie C, Fan Y, Huang Y, Wu S, Xu H, Liu L, et al. Class A1 scavenger receptors mediated macrophages in impaired intestinal barrier of inflammatory bowel disease. Annals of Translational Medicine. 2020;**8**(4):106

[37] Ito M, Suzuki H, Nakano N, Yamashita N, Sugiyama E, Maruyama M, et al. Superoxide anion and hydrogen peroxide release by macrophages from mice treated with Nocardia rubra cell-wall skeleton: Inhibition of macrophage cytotoxicity by a protease inhibitor but not by superoxide dismutase and catalase. Gann. 1983;**74**(1):128-136

[38] Jerkic M, Szaszi K, Laffey JG, Rotstein O, Zhang H. Key role of mesenchymal stromal cell interaction with macrophages in promoting repair of lung injury. International Journal of Molecular Sciences. 8 Feb 2023;**24**(4):3376

[39] Arabpour M, Saghazadeh A, Rezaei N. Anti-inflammatory and M2 macrophage polarization-promoting effect of mesenchymal stem cell-derived exosomes. International Immunopharmacology. 2021;**97**:107823

[40] Ding JY, Chen MJ, Wu LF, Shu GF, Fang SJ, Li ZY, et al. Mesenchymal stem cell-derived extracellular vesicles in skin wound healing: Roles, opportunities and challenges. Military Medical Research. 2023;**10**(1):36

[41] Weng YH, Chen WY, Lin YL, Wang JY, Chang MS. Blocking IL-19 signaling ameliorates allergen-induced airway inflammation. Frontiers in Immunology. 2019;**10**:968

[42] Molfino NA, Gossage D, Kolbeck R, Parker JM, Geba GP. Molecular and clinical rationale for therapeutic targeting of interleukin-5 and its receptor. Clinical and Experimental Allergy: Journal of the British Society for Allergy and Clinical Immunology. 2012;**42**(5):712-737

[43] Mai HL, Nguyen TVH, Bouchaud G, Henrio K, Cheminant MA, Magnan A, et al. Targeting the interleukin-7 receptor alpha by an anti-CD127 monoclonal antibody improves allergic airway inflammation in mice. Clinical and experimental allergy: Journal of the British Society for Allergy and Clinical Immunology. 2020;**50**(7):824-834

[44] Roussey JA, Viglianti SP, Teitz-Tennenbaum S, Olszewski MA, Osterholzer JJ. Anti-PD-1 antibody

treatment promotes clearance of persistent cryptococcal lung infection in mice. Journal of Immunology. 2017;**199**(10):3535-3546

[45] Verweyen EL, Schulert GS. Interfering with interferons: Targeting the JAK-STAT pathway in complications of systemic juvenile idiopathic arthritis (SJIA). Rheumatology (Oxford). 2022;**61**(3):926-935

[46] Hashimoto-Kataoka T, Hosen N, Sonobe T, Arita Y, Yasui T, Masaki T, et al. Interleukin-6/interleukin-21 signaling axis is critical in the pathogenesis of pulmonary arterial hypertension. Proceedings of the National Academy of Sciences of the United States of America. 2015;**112**(20):E2677-E2686

[47] Russo C, Colaianni V, Ielo G, Valle MS, Spicuzza L, Malaguarnera L. Impact of lung microbiota on COPD. Biomedicine. 6 Jun 2022;**10**(6):1337

[48] Eladham MW, Selvakumar B, Saheb Sharif-Askari N, Saheb Sharif-Askari F, Ibrahim SM, Halwani R. Unraveling the gut-lung axis: Exploring complex mechanisms in disease interplay. Heliyon. 2024;**10**(1):e24032

[49] Boyd RL, Fisher MJ, Jaeger MJ. Non-invasive lung function tests in rats with progressive papain-induced emphysema. Respiration Physiology. 1980;**40**(2):181-190

[50] Raub JA, Mercer RR, Miller FJ, Graham JA, O'Neil JJ. Dose response of elastase-induced emphysema in hamsters. The American Review of Respiratory Disease. 1982;**125**(4):432-435

[51] Wright JL, Churg A. Cigarette smoke causes physiologic and morphologic changes of emphysema in the guinea pig. The American Review of Respiratory Disease. 1990;**142**(6 Pt 1):1422-1428

[52] van der Strate BW, Postma DS, Brandsma CA, Melgert BN, Luinge MA, Geerlings M, et al. Cigarette smoke-induced emphysema: A role for the B cell? American Journal of Respiratory and Critical Care Medicine. 2006;**173**(7):751-758

[53] Wegmann M, Fehrenbach A, Heimann S, Fehrenbach H, Renz H, Garn H, et al. NO_2-induced airway inflammation is associated with progressive airflow limitation and development of emphysema-like lesions in C57bl/6 mice. Experimental and Toxicologic Pathology. 2005;**56**(6):341-350

[54] Tazaki G, Kondo T, Tajiri S, Tsuji C, Shioya S, Tanigaki T. Functional residual capacity and airway resistance in rats of COPD model induced by systemic hyaluronidase. The Tokai Journal of Experimental and Clinical Medicine. 2006;**31**(3):125-127

[55] Pera T, Zuidhof AB, Smit M, Menzen MH, Klein T, Flik G, et al. Arginaseinhibitionpreventsinflammation and remodeling in a guinea pig model of chronic obstructive pulmonary disease. The Journal of Pharmacology and Experimental Therapeutics. 2014;**349**(2):229-238

[56] Snider GL, Lucey EC, Faris B, Jung-Legg Y, Stone PJ, Franzblau C. Cadmium-chloride-induced air-space enlargement with interstitial pulmonary fibrosis is not associated with destruction of lung elastin. Implications for the pathogenesis of human emphysema. American Review in Respiratory Disease. 1988;**137**(4):918-923

[57] Taraseviciene-Stewart L, Douglas IS, Nana-Sinkam PS, Lee JD, Tuder RM, Nicolls MR, et al. Is alveolar destruction and emphysema in chronic obstructive pulmonary disease an immune disease?

Proceedings of the American Thoracic Society. 2006;**3**(8):687-690

[58] Morris DG, Huang X, Kaminski N, Wang Y, Shapiro SD, Dolganov G, et al. Loss of integrin alpha(v)beta6-mediated TGF-beta activation causes Mmp12-dependent emphysema. Nature. 2003;**422**(6928):169-173

[59] Baron RM, Choi AJ, Owen CA, Choi AM. Genetically manipulated mouse models of lung disease: Potential and pitfalls. American Journal of Physiology. Lung Cellular and Molecular Physiology. 2012;**302**(6):L485-L497

Chapter 3

Respiratory Surface Electromyography: Concepts, Utility, and Challenges

Kian Chung Ong

Abstract

In recent years, advancements in surface electromyography (EMG) have facilitated the monitoring and measurement of respiration in clinical medicine. Adapting and developing surface EMG (sEMG) specifically for assessing the muscles of respiration non-invasively, without the use of needles or catheters, heralds a new clinical dimension in evaluating respiratory symptomatology and pathophysiology. Surface EMG may be applied for the evaluation of the activity of the diaphragm and other muscles of respiration, such as the intercostal, sternocleidomastoid, and scalene muscles. This serves essential and complex functions for quantification of dyspnea, respiratory drive and effort, as well as for determining the onset of respiratory muscle fatigue. The potential uses for a portable, non-invasive, and preferably wireless respiratory surface EMG device are myriad. However, further applicability of respiratory surface EMG is hindered by technological issues, such as optimal EMG sensor designs and the requisite EMG signal conditioning for the evaluation of respiratory muscle activity. There is abundant scope and need for further collaborative research between clinicians and researchers. This chapter summarizes the basic concepts, uses, and challenges involved in the application of respiratory surface EMG, especially in patients with chronic respiratory disorders, such as pulmonary emphysema.

Keywords: dyspnea, respiratory drive, neural drive, respiratory effort, diaphragmatic function, respiratory function, monitoring, ventilation, sensor, review

1. Introduction

Electromyography (EMG) involves the acquisition of electrical signals produced by changes in action potentials of muscle units during muscular contraction and relaxation. This recording typically requires the placement of electrodes within or on the surface of the muscles of interest. The former type of EMG recording is invasive while the latter, also known as surface EMG (sEMG), is non-invasive and is generally the preferred mode for clinical purposes as well as for evaluation of exercise performance. The utility of sEMG is well established, and in recent years, its role in the evaluation of respiratory muscles is progressively recognized [1]. The commonest muscles of respiration that are used for respiratory sEMG are the diaphragm (that contributes to about 70% of the force of inspiration in healthy adults), intercostal,

IntechOpen

sternocleidomastoid, and scalene muscles. The field of respiratory sEMG is rapidly expanding and this chapter is aimed at exploring its role and potential, and the challenges faced in clinical application.

2. Rationale for respiratory sEMG

The respiratory neural drive is the efferent signal generated from the respiratory center to the respiratory muscles during inspiration [2], and this signal is generated in response to the myriad afferent sources that provide feedback to the respiratory control center in the body's respiratory control system. As illustrated in **Figure 1**, recording sEMG of respiratory muscles during inspiration provides a non-invasive and contemporaneous measurement of the respiratory neural drive [3]. Evaluating a subject's respiratory neural drive is important for two main reasons. The first is that it provides an objective and synchronic measure of the level of dyspnea the subject is experiencing. Since it is impossible to measure dyspneic sensation at the higher cortical centers currently, measuring the respiratory neural drive represents the best alternative, as the respiratory neural drive is an exact "copy" of the corollary discharge being sent to the higher cortical centers by the respiratory center after processing all the stimuli from afferent sources [4]. The second indication for measuring respiratory neural drive with respiratory sEMG is to non-invasively determine the intrathoracic pressures generated by the inspiratory pump, *P*mus.

2.1 Respiratory sEMG for evaluation of dyspnea

Previously, the ratio of the EMG amplitude of the diaphragm (EMGdi) during tidal breathing to the maximal volitional value (EMGdi/EMGdi, max) was proven as an index that provides the strongest correlation with dyspneic sensation in humans [5]. However, measurement of EMGdi requires the placement of an esophageal catheter containing multipaired electrodes, and as such, its measurement was confined

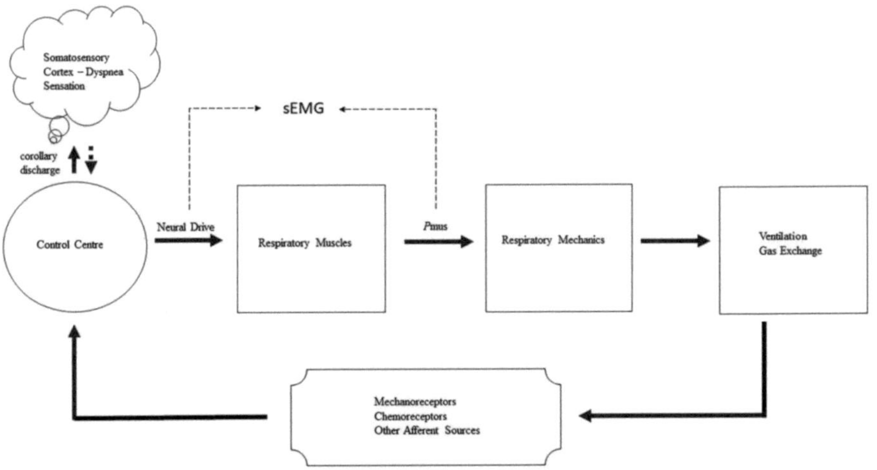

Figure 1.
A simplified illustration of the respiratory control feedback loop – thin dashed arrows represent signals that may be measured by sEMG. (Adapted from reference [3] with permission).

to research laboratories. The present developments in respiratory sEMG proffer a non-invasive biomarker of the sensation of dyspnea, and researchers have found the correlation between sEMG and transesophageal EMG of the diaphragm to be very high in stable patients with chronic obstructive pulmonary disease (COPD) undergoing treadmill exercise as well as in healthy subjects during inspiratory threshold loading [6, 7]. These researchers surmise that the sEMG percent maximum can serve as a non-invasive marker of neural respiratory drive. In patients presenting with acute heart failure, the severity of dyspnea is also found to correlate with sEMG activity of diaphragm and scalene muscles, the latter thus also providing a useful objective tool for assessment of dyspnea in non-respiratory conditions [8].

2.2 Respiratory sEMG for evaluation of respiratory effort

*P*mus is a function of the electric signal obtained from the sEMG of respiratory muscles, i.e., the sEMG correlates linearly or non-linearly with the *P*mus, with higher sEMG signal strengths corresponding to higher *P*mus. Therefore, respiratory sEMG provides a non-invasive means of estimating *P*mus. *P*mus is an indication of a subject's respiratory effort, a useful but oft inaccessible clinical parameter. Conventionally, the commonest way of determining *P*mus is by measuring the intrathoracic transpulmonary pressure generated during inspiration by the placement of an esophageal balloon or catheter (*P*es), which limits its clinical application to the intensive care unit (ICU) mainly. Researchers have recently attempted to establish an optimal electromechanical correlation of respiratory sEMG signals with *P*mus, thus decidedly simplifying and potentially broadening the scope of evaluating pulmonary mechanics in clinical practice [9]. Measuring *P*mus by sEMG, instead of *P*es, has an added advantage, especially in cases with minimal neuroventilatory uncoupling such as in healthy subjects or patients with mild COPD [3].

3. Current and potential clinical applications of respiratory sEMG

The global prevalence of COPD in 2020 was estimated to be 10.6%, or 480 million cases, and projected to increase to 600 million cases by 2050 [10]. Dyspnea or breathing discomfort and associated exercise limitation are the two most troubling symptoms reported by patients with COPD [11]. Accordingly, current global management guidelines on stable COPD prioritize the reduction of these symptoms as a key treatment goal [12]. However, as asserted in a comprehensive albeit lengthy dissertation on evaluating dyspnea in obstructive lung disease [3], the present methods of measuring dyspnea with questionnaires and symptom scores, i.e., by psychometric evaluation, are inadequate. This is especially so for the purpose of evaluating patient responses to treatments aimed at alleviating dyspnea. The lack of a universally accepted instrument for measuring dyspnea is testament to this inadequacy and the "profusion of measures" currently available, in fact, militates against progress in developing novel therapies for relief of dyspnea. Respiratory sEMG extends physiological assessment of dyspnea with a potential for widespread clinical application.

The health and societal burden inflicted by COPD is enormous, with healthcare resource utilization resulting from exacerbation of COPD accounting for most of the direct and indirect healthcare costs [10]. Clinical studies conducted in separate centers across the globe have found that adding sEMG measurement to current standard evaluation can meliorate the need for hospitalization and predict risk of readmissions following hospital discharge in patients with exacerbation of COPD [13–15]. COPD exacerbations have often been defined and treated according to clinical symptoms alone and not till recently has the addition of other objective parameters been recommended in grading the severity of such episodes for treatment purposes [12, 16]. The addition of sEMG, if widely available, will likely contribute to the evaluation and treatment of unstable COPD patients in future, as the foregoing clinical trials have shown. The benefits of sEMG can likewise be extended to respiratory monitoring of any case of acute dyspnea. The recent finding of *P*mus as the parameter that best predicts success of non-invasive ventilation and high-flow oxygen therapy in patients with COVID-19 infection serves to emphasize the need to measure *P*mus, reliably and readily, in conscious patients during acute situations [17]. The recent pandemic has also highlighted the requisition for accurate respiratory assessment of patients on remote telemonitoring [18]. The availability and portability of respiratory surface EMG equipment will undoubtedly contribute to the accuracy of respiratory monitoring in numerous scenarios in future.

In addition to the usefulness of respiratory sEMG based on its amplitude correlation with respiratory neural drive and respiratory effort as explicated above, another

Uses of respiratory sEMG or EMGdi
• Monitoring respiratory effort during sleep studies*
• Intensive care—optimizing patient and ventilator interaction*
• Assess the severity and/or predict treatment response and safe discharge in exacerbation of COPD and heart failure*
• Predict success or failure of non-invasive ventilation/oxygen therapy in acute respiratory failure*
• Evaluation of asthma in children*
• Monitoring of respiration in infants*
• Correlation with dyspnea during exercise in healthy subjects, COPD and heart failure patients*
• Correlation with chronic dyspnea during activities of daily living
• Approval for "relief of dyspnoea" indication of interventions by approving authorities
• Evaluation of dyspnea during exercise testing in athletes and in patients with cardiopulmonary disorders
• Exercise prescription for healthy subjects (with ventilatory limitation of exercise) and patients with cardiopulmonary disorders
• Breathing training/retraining during chest physiotherapy and cardiopulmonary rehabilitation
• Evaluation of response to cardiopulmonary rehabilitation
• Evaluation and treatment of psychogenic dyspnea/ hyperventilation
• Determine the onset of diaphragmatic muscle fatigue during exertion in acute/chronic conditions
• Telemonitoring and follow-up of patients
• Regulating support of home ventilators in chronic respiratory failure
• Evaluation and training for vocalization/singing
• Biofeedback for Yoga, relaxation exercises, and meditation
• Enhancing exercise performance—including gymnastics, swimming, diving, and outdoor sports
• Supplementary mobile health device

**Asterisks indicate published studies are available.*

Table 1.
Current and potential uses of respiratory sEMG or EMGdi.

functional dimension is the potential of EMG in detecting muscle fatigue [19]. This is made possible by identifying changes in the frequency of EMG signals with the onset of muscle fatigue, thus generating possibilities beyond current capabilities in exercise testing and prescription [3, 20].

A list of the current and potential applications of respiratory surface EMG is presented in **Table 1**.

4. Challenges in developing respiratory sEMG

The transition of theoretical concepts of respiratory sEMG to practical usage is not straightforward. The technological challenges of sEMG may be classified into two—signal acquisition and signal conditioning [21]. The former requires optimal sensor design and placement, as sEMG signals are generally weak (measured in microvolts) and have high signal-to-noise ratios. This is especially applicable in relation to surface EMG sensors for respiratory muscles like the diaphragm, as high impedance due to overlying tissues and "cross-talk" from surrounding muscles is encountered. sEMG signal processing is correspondingly not a simple matter—signal amplification, noise reduction, and signal interpretation require complex algorithms, especially if precise electromechanical association is desired, e.g., in correlating sEMG signals with respiratory parameters like *P*mus, breath flow rate, tidal volume, etc. Further progress is imminent as an important initial step appears to have been set in motion with the recent round-table discussion among interested researchers focusing on standardization and developing best practices in the analysis and applications of respiratory sEMG [22].

5. Conclusion

The use of non-invasive sEMG for the measurement and monitoring of respiratory muscle activity portends a promising new paradigm in the subjective and objective assessment of breathing. The clinical potential of respiratory sEMG in the management of patients with dyspnea, a symptom *sine qua non* of COPD, is immense.

Conflict of interest

The author declares no conflict of interest.

Author details

Kian Chung Ong
Chestmed Private Limited, Mount Elizabeth Medical Centre, Singapore

*Address all correspondence to: ongkc@chestmed.com.sg

References

[1] van Leuteren RW, Hutten GJ, de Waal CG, Dixon P, van Kaam AH, de Jongh FH. Processing transcutaneous electromyography measurements of respiratory muscles, a review of analysis techniques. Journal of Electromyography and Kinesiology. 2019;**48**:176-186. DOI: 10.1016/j.jelekin.2019.07.014

[2] Jolley CJ, Luo YM, Steier J, et al. Neural respiratory drive in healthy subjects and in COPD. The European Respiratory Journal. 2009;**33**(2): 289-297. DOI: 10.1183/09031936.00093408

[3] Ong KC. Clinical evaluation of dyspnoea in obstructive lung disease – Progressing from psychometrics to physiology. Medical Research Archives. 2024;**12**(2):1-12. DOI: 10.18103/mra.v12i2.5019

[4] Laviolette L, Laveneziana P; ERS Research Seminar Faculty. Dyspnoea: A multidimensional and multidisciplinary approach. The European Respiratory Journal. 2014;**43**(6):1750-1762. DOI:10.1183/09031936.00092613

[5] O'Donnell DE, Milne KM, James MD, de Torres JP, Neder JA. Dyspnea in COPD: New mechanistic insights and management implications. Advances in Therapy. 2020;**37**(1):41-60. DOI: 10.1007/s12325-019-01128-9

[6] Wu W, Guan L, Li X, et al. Correlation and compatibility between surface respiratory electromyography and transesophageal diaphragmatic electromyography measurements during treadmill exercise in stable patients with COPD. International Journal of Chronic Obstructive Pulmonary Disease. 2017;**12**:3273-3280. DOI: 10.2147/COPD.S148980

[7] Lin L, Guan L, Wu W, Chen R. Correlation of surface respiratory electromyography with esophageal diaphragm electromyography. Respiratory Physiology & Neurobiology. 2019;**259**:45-52. DOI: 10.1016/j.resp.2018.07.004

[8] Luiso D, Villanueva JA, Belarte-Tornero LC, et al. Surface respiratory electromyography and dyspnea in acute heart failure patients. PLoS One. 2020;**15**(4):e0232225. DOI: 10.1371/journal.pone.0232225

[9] Graßhoff J, Petersen E, Farquharson F, et al. Surface EMG-based quantification of inspiratory effort: A quantitative comparison with P_{es}. Critical Care. 2021;**25**(1):441. DOI: 10.1186/s13054-021-03833-w

[10] Boers E, Barrett M, Su JG, et al. Global burden of chronic obstructive pulmonary disease through 2050. JAMA Network Open. 2023;**6**(12):e2346598. DOI: 10.1001/jamanetworkopen.2023.46598

[11] Svedsater H, Roberts J, Patel C, Macey J, Hilton E, Bradshaw L. Life impact and treatment preferences of individuals with asthma and chronic obstructive pulmonary disease: Results from qualitative interviews and focus groups. Advances in Therapy. 2017;**34**(6):1466-1481. DOI: 10.1007/s12325-017-0557-0

[12] Agustí A, Celli BR, Criner GJ, et al. Global initiative for chronic obstructive lung disease 2023 report: GOLD executive summary. The European Respiratory Journal. 2023;**61**(4):2300239. DOI: 10.1183/13993003.00239-2023

[13] Zhang DD, Lu G, Zhu XF, et al. Neural respiratory drive measured

using surface electromyography of diaphragm as a physiological biomarker to predict hospitalization of acute exacerbation of chronic obstructive pulmonary disease patients. Chinese Medical Journal. 2018;**131**(23):2800-2807. DOI: 10.4103/0366-6999.246057

[14] Murphy PB, Kumar A, Reilly C, et al. Neural respiratory drive as a physiological biomarker to monitor change during acute exacerbations of COPD. Thorax. 2011;**66**(7):602-608. DOI: 10.1136/thx.2010.151332

[15] Suh ES, Mandal S, Harding R, et al. Neural respiratory drive predicts clinical deterioration and safe discharge in exacerbations of COPD. Thorax. 2015;**70**(12):1123-1130. DOI: 10.1136/thoraxjnl-2015-207188

[16] Celli BR, Fabbri LM, Aaron SD, et al. An updated definition and severity classification of chronic obstructive pulmonary disease exacerbations: The Rome proposal. American Journal of Respiratory and Critical Care Medicine. 2021;**204**(11):1251-1258. DOI: 10.1164/rccm.202108-1819PP

[17] Crimi C, Murphy P, Patout M, Sayas J, Winck JC. Lessons from COVID-19 in the management of acute respiratory failure. Breathe (Sheffield, England). 2023;**19**(1):230035. DOI: 10.1183/20734735.0035-2023

[18] Ten Broeke CEM, Himmelreich JCL, Cals JWL, Lucassen WAM, Harskamp RE. The Roth score as a triage tool for detecting hypoxaemia in general practice: A diagnostic validation study in patients with possible COVID-19. Primary Health Care Research & Development. 2021;**22**:e56. DOI: 10.1017/S1463423621000347

[19] Ertl P, Kruse A, Tilp M. Detecting fatigue thresholds from electromyographic signals: A systematic review on approaches and methodologies. Journal of Electromyography and Kinesiology. 2016;**30**:216-230. DOI: 10.1016/j.jelekin.2016.08.002

[20] Cavalcanti JD, Fregonezi GAF, Sarmento AJ, et al. Electrical activity and fatigue of respiratory and locomotor muscles in obstructive respiratory diseases during field walking test. PLoS One. 2022;**17**(4):e0266365. DOI: 10.1371/journal.pone.0266365

[21] Gao S et al. Use of advanced materials and artificial intelligence in electromyography signal detection and interpretation. Advanced Intelligent Systems. 2022;**4**(10):2200063. DOI: 10.1002/aisy.202200063

[22] Jonkman AH, Warnaar RSP, Baccinelli W, et al. Analysis and applications of respiratory surface EMG: Report of a round table meeting. Critical Care. 2024;**28**(1):2. DOI: 10.1186/s13054-023-04779-x

Chapter 4

Overview of Bronchoscopy and Its Employment in Pulmonary Emphysema

Ola Arab and Lana Kourieh

Abstract

Bronchoscopy is a medical procedure usually performed by a specialist for diagnostic or therapeutic purposes in the airway passages. There are two main types of procedure: rigid and flexible bronchoscopy, in addition to developed types such as ultrasound and navigational bronchoscopy to help improve the required outcome. There are several indications for bronchoscopy, but the leading one is suspicion of lung cancer, followed by detection of possible pulmonary infection. On the other hand, hypoxia is the main contraindication for his operation. A precise clinical history of the patient should be taken and multiple tests should be provided before the procedure. Sampling can be done in different ways depending on the indication. Overall, bronchoscopy is a minimum invasive procedure and complications are uncommon, especially for highly experienced doctors. However, patients with chronic pulmonary disorders such as COPD patients must be handled cautiously, especially when treated under sedation and those who have exacerbations.

Keywords: bronchoscopy, endobronchial ultrasound, navigational bronchoscopy, indications, contraindications, bronchoscopy procedure, COPD, safety

1. Introduction

Bronchoscopy is the procedure of passing a camera or telescope into the trachea reaching the lower respiratory tracts to examine the large and medium-sized airways. It may be performed either in the way preferred by physicians where the patient is under local anesthetic with or without sedation using a flexible scope or as surgeons usually do, under general anesthesia with a rigid scope [1].

Bronchoscopy procedure has become a major tool for the pulmonologist, in addition to its diagnostic applications from airway inspection to sampling, it has also been used for its therapeutic capabilities such as palliative treatment of endobronchial tumors, also in the treatment of asthma and emphysema [2].

IntechOpen

2. Types of bronchoscopy

There are two main types of bronchoscopy procedure: Rigid bronchoscopy and flexible bronchoscopy.

2.1 Rigid bronchoscope

A rigid bronchoscope is a stainless steel, straight cylindrical tube with an external diameter of 9–14 mm (Adult scopes are usually 7–9 mm and pediatric scopes are 3.5–6 mm). The length of the bronchoscope can be up to 45 cm and the thickness of walls is 2–3 mm. The tube is hollowed to allow the passage of different tools. The proximal third of some rigid bronchoscopes can have several ports for lung ventilation when inserted into the main stem bronchus (**Figure 1**) [4, 5].

Visualization *via* a rigid bronchoscope can be done directly through the hollowed tube of the scope which is limited and unsuitable for fine details, or can be done by using a rigid optic telescope or video scope that is passed through the scope which is more convenient [6].

2.2 Flexible bronchoscope

A flexible bronchoscope is basically a thin flexible tube with a diameter range of 2.2–6.3 mm, containing fiberoptic bundles that carry light to the distal end inside the airways and transmit the image to an eyepiece or a monitor chip (video bronchoscope) which are more suitable for teaching and observation by multiple physicians. The flexible bronchoscope is also equipped with channels to insert different tools (brush, biopsy forceps, transbronchial aspiration needles, etc.) (**Figure 2**). An important advantage of this bronchoscope is the rotation of the distal end 180–180 degrees *via* a lever at the handle end of the scope in addition to manual wrist rotation which facilitates airway examination [2].

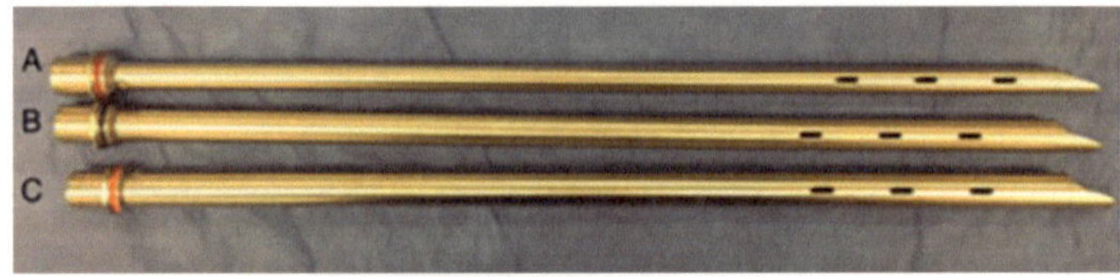

Figure 1.
The three most common sizes of bronchial tubes are used in adults: (outer diameter/inner diameter mm color) A. 10/9.2 mm red, B. 12/11 mm (black), and C. 13.2/12.2 mm (orange) [3].

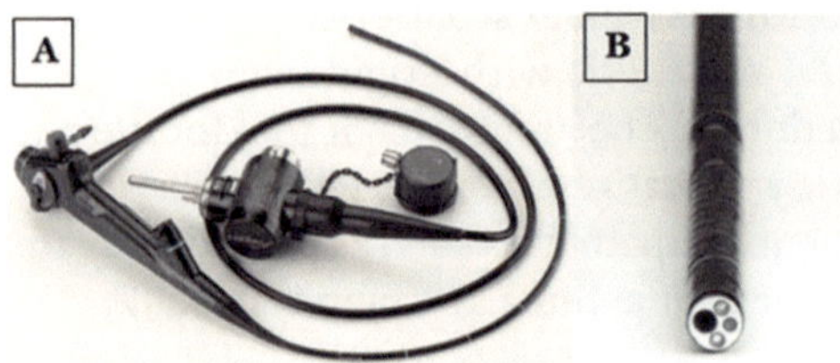

Figure 2.
A. Video flexible bronchoscope with connections to image processor and light source. B. Distal end of a video bronchoscope showing the instrument channel, fiberoptic, and charge-coupled device video chip that connects to the monitor for image processing [2].

There are three main sizes of flexible bronchoscope [6]:

- *Pediatric (Ultrathin) bronchoscope* with an outer diameter of 2.8 mm and a channel width of 1.2 mm. This small size allows suctioning and passing small tools such as brush for cytology tests and biopsy forceps. Nevertheless, clear visualization is limited to small sizes.
- *Adult (Standard) bronchoscope* has an outer diameter of 4.9–5.5 mm and a channel size of 2 mm, which allows baskets and greater suctioning.
- *Therapeutic bronchoscopes* of an external diameter of 6–6.2 mm and a larger channel size of 2.8–3.2 mm. This size is used for laser therapy and insertion of electrocautery instruments.

Over the recent decades, two new bronchoscopy techniques have been developed to help biopsy mediastinal and peripheral pulmonary lesions and examine beyond the airways.

2.2.1 Endobronchial ultrasound (EBUS)

The flexible bronchoscope in this type of bronchoscopy, the probe is combined with an ultrasound probe at the distal end of the scope, which allows the examiner to view more extended bronchial structures, lymph nodes, masses, and mediastinal structures. There are two types of the EBUS scope:

- *Radial probe*: This scope was developed first for early evaluation and detection of infiltrated cancer in the airway tissue, as well as an examination of peripheral and mediastinal lymph nodes [7–9]. The radial probe can be in two forms [10]:
    - *The miniature:* The probe is equipped with a balloon-tipped catheter that inflates with saline to obtain clear visualization by optimizing contact between airway walls and probe (**Figure 3**).
    - *The ultra-miniature:* In this type the inserted probe is covered with a guiding sheath, the lesion is examined and the image is obtained. Then the probe is removed with the sheath remaining in the spot and a biopsy forceps or a brush is passed to the sheath location for sampling (**Figure 4**).
- *Convex probe:* This scope allows direct visualization during biopsy sampling. The scope is equipped with a convex transducer at the tip that scans parallelly to the insertion direction of the bronchoscope (**Figure 4**). A saline inflatable balloon is also combined for a clear image and a fine aspirating needle covered with a removable sheath is inserted through the working channel to the lesion site for sampling during visualization [10, 11].

2.2.2 Electromagnetic navigational bronchoscopy (ENB)

This technology was first commercially available in 2006, where bronchoscopy is combined and compassed with CT imaging, which allows biopsy of lesions that can be difficult to reach [12]. It is usually performed in two stages: the planning stage and the procedure stage.

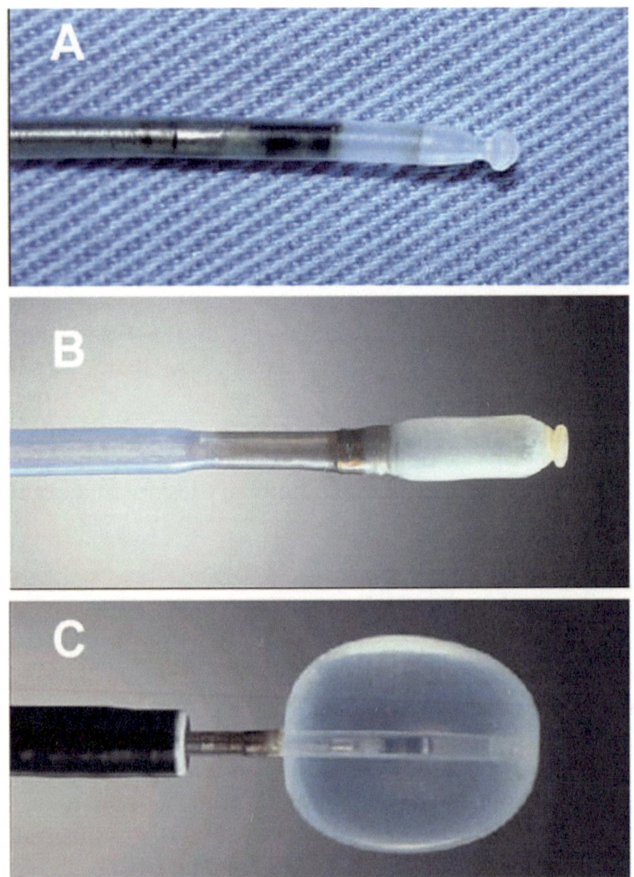

Figure 3.
A: miniature radial probe, B: balloon tip catheter, and C: the balloon tip inflated with saline [10].

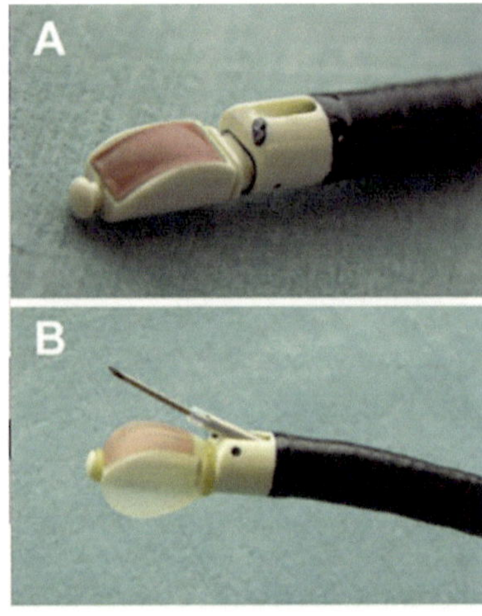

Figure 4.
A: miniature radial probe, B: the balloon tip inflated with saline and a fine needle is inserted for transbronchial aspiration [10].

In the planning stage, the patient goes through a thin slice CT scan, which is then uploaded to the computer software that provides a three-dimensional image of the bronchial tree with more than one highlighted pathway created to the lesion for better biopsy outcome.

For the procedure stage, the patient is laid on an electromagnetic mat under their chest which is registered with both; the therapeutic bronchoscope and the three-dimensional airway construction with the highlighted pathways [13].

The disadvantage of this technology compared to the traditional CT-guided biopsy is the additional exposure to radiation for the planning stage and the cost of the dedicated software. However, with very minimum complications [14].

3. Indications for bronchoscopy

The major indications for bronchoscopy are suspicion of lung cancer followed by suspicion of pulmonary infection for microbiological sampling [2]. **Table 1** lists the main indications for bronchoscopy, including diagnostic and therapeutic purposes.

4. Contraindications of bronchoscopy

- The main contraindication for bronchoscopy is hypoxia which cannot be adequately corrected by oxygen supplementation. Therefore, if the patient's air saturation is less than 90% at rest or less than 8 kPa, the risk of hypoxia is greatly increased during the procedure [1, 2].

Diagnostic indications	*Investigation of symptoms* like persistent cough, hemoptysis, and recurrent infection.
	Suspected lung cancer: Patients who have one or more of these signs: unexplained paralysis of vocal cords, stridor, localized monophonic wheeze, unexplained paralysis of hemi-diaphragm or raised right hemi-diaphragm and unexplained pleural effusions.
	Assessment of nodules or masses identified on radiology.
	Staging of lung cancer
	Suspected pulmonary infection: Assessment of pulmonary infiltrates, identification of organisms.
	Differential cell counts and cytology
	Transbronchial lung biopsy
Therapeutic indications	Foreign body removal
	Clearance of airway secretions
	Recurring mucus obstruction that causes lobar collapse and lung atelectasis in patients on ventilators.
	Emphysema (endobronchial lung volume reduction)
	Bronchial thermoplasty for asthma
	Endobronchial ablation of tumor (cryotherapy, electrocautery, laser).
	Insertion of airway stents.

Table 1.
Indications for bronchoscopy [1, 2].

- If the forced expiratory volume (FEV1) was below 40% [1].
- Bleeding tendency: Blood clotting abnormalities, especially platelet level <50,000/mm3 [1].
- Pulmonary hypertension (PHT), uremia, superior vena cava obstruction (SVCO), liver disease, and immunosuppression [1].
- Recent myocardial infarction (MI) may be associated with cardiac ischemia during bronchoscopy [1].
- Cervical spine instability [3].
- Failure of the patient or his representative (in special cases) to provide consent for the operation [2].

However, even in these circumstances, similar to other invasive procedures, firm cut-offs are not given as the risks and benefits of bronchoscopy should be carefully evaluated on an individual patient basis [2, 3].

5. Patient preparation and procedure

5.1 Patient preparation

5.1.1 Information

Informed consent should be obtained from the patient or the patient's health care power of attorney, ideally >24 h prior to the procedure [1, 15]. The patient should be provided with written information in advance of the procedure and the key aspects, such as the risks of the procedure and the effects of any sedation and possible complications. Also, alternative approaches should be discussed before final consent [1, 2].

5.1.2 Clinical history

- A focused history and physical examination should be obtained to ensure the procedure is clinically indicated. The patients should fast (nothing by mouth) for six to eight hours before the procedure, but they may be allowed to drink water for up to 2 hours before the procedure [2, 15].
- Patients should have a full blood count and clotting prior to transbronchial lung biopsy and interventional procedures, such as tumor ablation [2].
- It is safe to stop anticoagulation if a patient is taking aspirin or prophylactic low-molecular-weight-heparin LMWh. On the other hand, patient should stop clopidogrel seven days before the procedure (may require cardiology consultation), also the patient should wait until INr is below 1.5 if he is on warfarin, in high-risk conditions, for example, mitral prosthetic metal valve, prosthetic valve or thrombophilia syndromes the patient may need a full-dose of LMWh on days before bronchoscopy [1].

- Besides tests, an ECG may be performed in patients with a history of cardiac disease. Blood sugar should be checked in patients with diabetes [1].

- Before starting the procedure, oxygen saturation level should be monitored using pulse oximetry, also intravenous access should be assured. The patient's medication list, any possible allergies, and all laboratory results should be checked [15].

- Pulse oximetry should be monitored during the procedure and venous access should be present in all patients [1].

- Spirometry should be used if oxygen saturation is below 95% [2].

- Arterial blood gas test should be done if oxygen saturation is below 92% [2].

5.1.3 Sedation

Most bronchoscopy procedures are performed under moderate conscious sedation even though the procedure may be performed without sedation. The sedatives used are usually chosen based on the clinician's preference (e.g., benzodiazepines, opioids, and dexmedetomidine). There are some cases where procedures may require more deep sedation or general anesthesia. In general, physicians should be aware of the potential side effects and how to manage patients receiving these medications regardless of the sedation or anesthesia used. If patients are to have any sedation, it is highly important that someone is going to accompany them home after the procedure [2].

- *Nebulized bronchodilators* are considered if there is evidence of bronchospasm in patients with asthma [1, 2].

- *Prophylactic antibiotics* are considered if there is a very high risk of endocarditis: asplenia, heart valve prosthesis, or previous history of endocarditis [2].

5.1.4 Procedure

The procedure can be performed with the patient sitting upright in a semi-recumbent position and being approached from the front (**Figure 5A**). This has the advantage of allowing it to be carried out in sicker patients who are desaturated upon lying flat [2].

The posterior approach with the patient lying flat is also widely used (**Figure 5B**). This approach is also required in several procedures such as endobronchial ultrasound and the super dimension procedure [2].

The nasal route is the most accessible way to the trachea where the bronchoscope is introduced into the nasal cavity, as this route gives more stability when taking biopsies and it permits the patient to cough and spit out secretions more easily. When the nasal way is not possible, a mouth guard is used and advanced to the level of the vocal cords [1, 15].

During the procedure, the movement and the appearance of the vocal cords are assessed. Later, while the bronchoscope advances beyond the vocal cords, a careful inspection of the entire airway is performed. Assessment of any abnormal endobronchial lesions or mucosal abnormalities, as well as any evidence of narrowing or dynamic collapse, is done particularly [15].

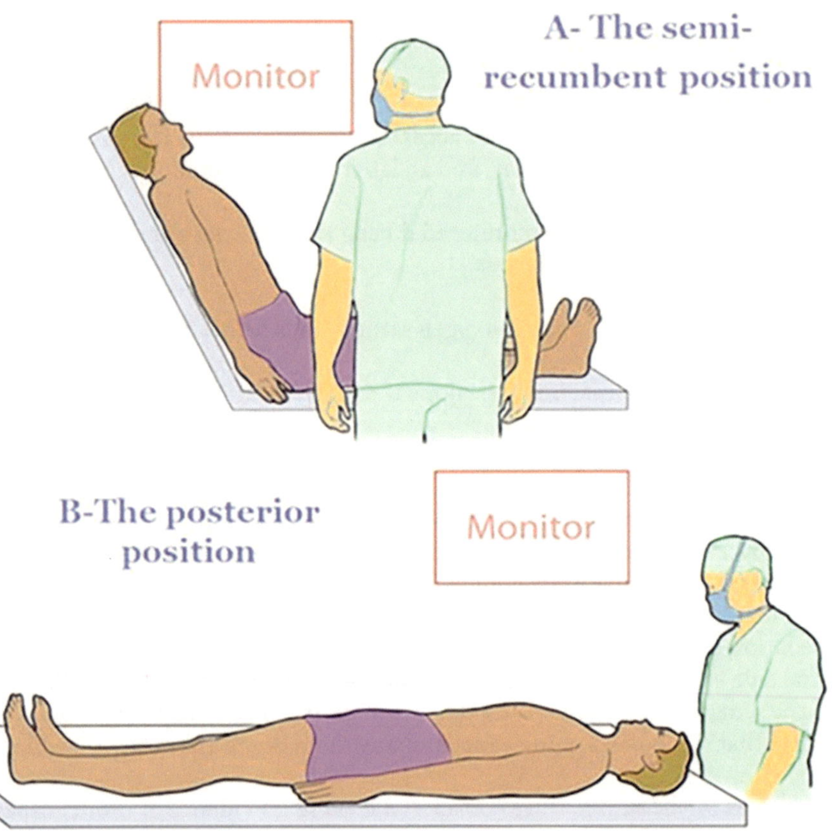

Figure 5.
Patient positioning during bronchoscopy procedure: A: The semi-recumbent position, B: The posterior position.

All sections of the bronchial tree should be visually checked, including the cords and trachea. Also, to increase the diagnostic yield of bronchoscopy in lung cancer suspected cases, a chest X-ray or CT may help to localize the area of concern, so the biopsy site can then be targeted accurately [1].

It is preferable to record photos and videos so they can be used as references when it is needed. Any unnecessary contact with the mucosa should be avoided to stay away from any available trauma, also unnecessary suction should be avoided, as this can increase hypoxia [1, 15].

The appropriate tools for the procedure are chosen according to the required indication and the task to be performed during bronchoscopy, such as tumor debulking or taking a tissue biopsy. At the end of the procedure, a final evaluation of the airway should be performed to ensure adequate hemostasis. The patient may need a chest X-ray after the procedure to evaluate the presence of a pneumothorax. All patients should be monitored before, during, and after bronchoscopy. The patient may be discharged on the same day after ensuring recovery and the absence of any complications, also an appointment is scheduled to follow up on the case. Since the effect of medications may last for several hours, the patient is advised not to drive, operate heavy machinery, or participate in any activity that requires full consciousness for the rest of the day [15].

DOI: http://dx.doi.org/10.5772/intechopen.1004525

6. Sampling in bronchoscopy

Different sampling techniques can be performed based on indication and the required test [2]:

- *Bronchial washings (BW):* This technique allows targeted sampling of proximal or segmental airways. The bronchoscope is held proximal and close to the location of abnormality. An aliquot of 10–20 mL saline is instilled and aspirated back. The sensitivity of bronchial washings is very variable (average 50%; range 21–76%).

- *Endobronchial biopsy (EBB):* In this technique, forceps are inserted through the instrument channel of the bronchoscope. The forceps are just opened, at the location of the lesion and then closed in order to obtain biopsies under direct vision (**Figure 6**). Multiple biopsies are recommended for more accurate results.

- *Bronchial brushings (BB):* This sample can be obtained by using the cytology brush to scrape some cells from the surface of the lesion or the examined area. The brush consists of fine bristles with a protective plastic sheath. The instrument is passed through the instrument channel of the bronchoscope toward the abnormal area. The sheath is then removed and the brush is rubbed against the abnormal mucosa. The brush is then withdrawn back into the plastic sheath (**Figure 7**).

- *Bronchoalveolar lavage (BAL):* The technique is performed by wedging the bronchoscope on the desired subsegment. With the bronchoscope in position, saline aliquots of 50 ml are repeatedly instilled and aspirated either manually or using a low-pressure suction, reaching a total of 250 ml based on the desired testing or indication.

- *Transbronchial biopsy (TBB):* This technique is performed to evaluate the assessment of diffuse lung disease and in patients where there is a localized parenchymal shadow. The biopsy forceps are inserted into the desired segment through the instrument channel of the bronchoscope. The insertion of the

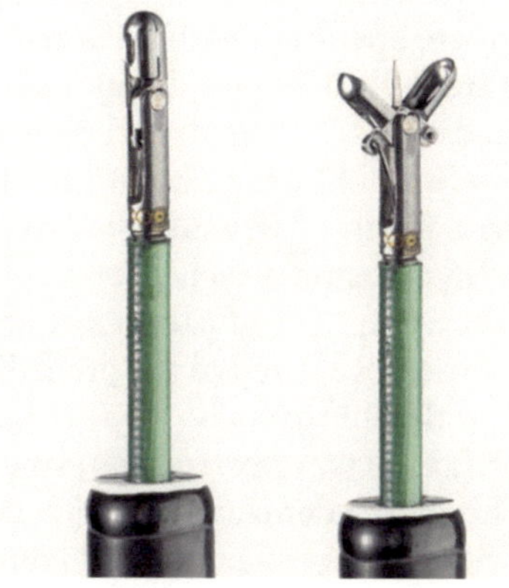

Figure 6.
Distal view of the biopsy forceps in an open and closed position [2].

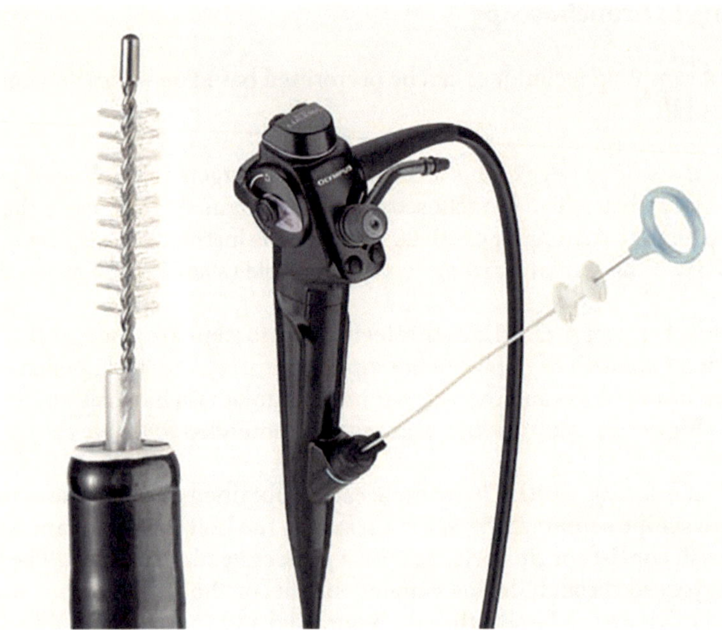

Figure 7.
Close-up of a bronchial brush (left) and handle (right): when the brush is pulled out of the sheath [2].

forceps proceeds until resistance is felt during inspiration. The forceps are then withdrawn 1–2 cm and opened. At this point, the patient should breathe out whilst the forceps are moved further during expiration. When resistance is felt, the forceps are closed and gently pulled. It is recommended to obtain multiple biopsies for better outcome.

7. Complications of bronchoscopy

7.1 Complications of flexible bronchoscopy

Flexible bronchoscopy is a safe operation with a low rate of complications. Reported mortality rates in large series are 0.01–0.04% and major complications of 0.08–1.1% [1]. In a recent study performed on 3,473 patients had done FB. Complications occurred in 5.3% of patients were as follows: 2.2% suffered from moderate to severe bleeding, 0.7% had pneumothorax, and 0.8% suffered from severe bronchospasm. Generally, complications like (hypoxemia, psychomotor agitation, arrhythmias, vomiting, or hypotension), were shown in 1.6% of patients; and cardiopulmonary arrest occurred in 0.03% of them. No deaths related to the procedures were recorded [16].

In general, complications of flexible bronchoscopy consist of respiratory depression, pneumonia, pneumothorax, airway obstruction, laryngospasm, cardiopulmonary arrest, arrhythmias, pulmonary edema, vasovagal episodes, fever (especially following BAL), septicemia, hemorrhage, nausea, and vomiting [1].

Although most complications are caused by sedation and topical anesthesia [17]. However, several factors also play a role in causing complications, including the patient's clinical condition, the insertion of the bronchoscope into the airway, in addition to the techniques used in taking biopsies such as BAL, EBB, TBB, and BB [18, 19]. Usually, most complications occur within 2 h after the procedure, and only a minority of patients require hospitalization [17, 20–22]. In general, side effects such as tension pneumothorax, heart/respiratory failure, and death are rare but they are serious and require interrupting the operation. The previous side effects are often related to the severity of underlying heart or lung disease, as well as to severe central airway obstruction [21, 23, 24].

To ensure the lowest rate of complications, standardized care protocols are developed, in addition to continuing suitable training of specialist doctors and nursing staff [16].

Moderate-to-severe bleeding occurs in 70.7% of patients, as a result of mechanical trauma from the bronchoscope, suctioning, brushing, or sampling, but is more common with transbronchial lung biopsy (TBB) (1.6–4.4%). The patient clinical status also plays a role, as patients suffering from malignancy, immunocompromise, or uremia are more susceptible to bleeding [1].

In cases where severe hemorrhage occurs, the patient should be turned onto the side of the bleeding to protect the other lung. The bleeding area may be tamponade using a balloon-tipped vascular catheter. If bleeding continues, emergency interventional radiology or thoracic surgery may be recommended [1].

7.2 Complications of rigid bronchoscopy

Similar to flexible bronchoscopy, when rigid bronchoscopy is performed by well-trained doctors, complications are uncommon [25]. The most common complaint following rigid bronchoscopy is a sore throat, which usually subsides 24–48 hours after the procedure. As for serious complications, they are uncommon (<2%) and their causes are limited to either anesthesia or the operation itself [26, 27].

Several studies confirmed the rarity of complications, one of which took place in a tertiary-care university hospital, the study included 775 rigid bronchoscopies, the overall complication rate was 13.4%, most of the complications were mild, and severe complications were rare with a 0.4% mortality rate [28–30]. Another large series included 11,000 rigid bronchoscopies, and only 2 deaths were recorded [31, 32]. As for therapeutic applications, a recent study of the AQuIRE registry found the overall complication rate of therapeutic bronchoscopy done with rigid bronchoscopy to be 3.4% [32, 33].

Injury to the oropharyngeal structures, laryngeal edema, spinal cord injury, injury to vocal cords and arytenoids, airway laceration and perforation, and hypoxemia-induced cardiac ischemia and arrhythmias [3] are serious complications of rigid bronchoscopy that could be avoided with proper preoperative assessment, appropriate instrument preparation and maintain adequate communication with the anesthesiologist [28].

8. Bronchoscopy safety in patients with chronic obstructive pulmonary disease (COPD)

Although bronchoscopy is considered as a minimum invasive procedure, the British Thoracic Society has listed patients with COPD who need diagnostic bronchoscopy as a needing caution. A study by Grendelmeier *et al.* reported no difference in bronchoscopy complications between COPD and non-COPD patients [34]. On the other hand, a study conducted by Bellinger *et al.*, to compare complications rate between patients with or without COPD going through bronchoscopy procedure under moderate sedation; concluded that bronchoscopy is generally tolerable with few complications in patients with COPD. However, those with confirmed severe/ very severe COPD are at higher risk of complications than those without COPD [35]. Also, a systematic review and meta-analysis on the topic reported that the major complications rate in bronchoscopy are higher in COPD patients with exacerbations than those who are stable [36].

9. Bronchoscopic management of emphysema

Recently, several bronchoscopy techniques have been used for intervention in chronic pulmonary diseases such as emphysema. The main objective of such procedures is to deflate the volume of the lung or the targeted lobe, which can be done with one of the following techniques [37]:

- *Endobronchial valves:*

  Valves in those techniques are essentially one-way valves that are introduced into a segmental targeted lobe *via* bronchoscopy with a flexible catheter under local or general anesthesia. Those valves facilitate the expiration of trapped air in the targeted lobe and prevent air inspiration, therefore preventing lobar or lung collapse. Recent RCTs concluded that misplacement of valves or patients on collateral ventilation do not come with promising results. Therefore, endobronchial valves are recommended in either heterogenous or homogenous emphysema patients without collateral ventilation, with the assessment of CT scan along with using the Chartis system for endobronchial measuring [37–39].

- *Endobronchial coils:*

  Endobronchial coils are nickel-titanium shape-memory coils that are introduced into subsegmental bronchi in a targeted lobe *via* bronchoscopy with an insertion catheter. These coils retract the parenchyma, decrease lung volume, and facilitate lung rebound. The procedure is performed with fluoroscopy guidance under general anesthesia. About 10–12 coils are placed in the upper lobes and up to 14 in the lower lobe. Usually, treatment of the other side must be performed after 1–3 months from the first side treatment. Unlike endobronchial valves and according to recent studies, this technique is recommended for heterogeneous or homogenous emphysema patients with or without collateral ventilation. However, this technique cannot be performed when the lungs are over-destroyed because viable parenchyma is required for enhanced performance [37, 39–41].

- *Bronchial thermal vapor ablation:*

  In this technique, a hot water steam is delivered through a bronchoscopic catheter to a targeted area of the lung, which causes parenchymal tissue fibrosis due to inflammation caused by heat and eventually lung volume reduction. This procedure is performed for heterogeneous emphysema patients with or without collateral ventilation [37, 39, 42].

Author details

Ola Arab* and Lana Kourieh
Department of Biochemistry and Microbiology, College of Pharmacy, Aleppo University, Aleppo, Syria

*Address all correspondence to: ola93arab@hotmail.com

References

[1] Chapman S, Robinson G, Stradling J, West S, Wrightson J. Oxford Handbook of Respiratory Medicine. 3rd ed. United Kingdom: Oxford University Press; 2014. p. 906. ISBN 0198703864, 9780198703860

[2] Shah P. Atlas of Flexible Bronchoscopy. 1st ed. United States: CRC Press; 2011. p. 256. ISBN 034096832X, 9780340968321

[3] Batra H, Yarmus L. Indications and complications of rigid Bronchoscopy. Expert Review of Respiratory Medicine. 2018;**12**(6):509-520. DOI: 10.1080/17476348.2018.1473037

[4] Ayers ML, Beamis JF Jr. Rigid bronchoscopy in the twenty-first century. Clinics in Chest Medicine. 2001;**22**(2):355-364. DOI: 10.1016/s0272-5231(05)70049-6

[5] Nicastri DG, Weiser TS. Rigid bronchoscopy: Indications and techniques. Operative Techniques in Thoracic Cardiovascular Surgery. 2012;**17**:44-51. DOI: 10.1053/j.optechstcvs.2012.03.001

[6] Paradis TJ, Dixon J, Tieu BH. The role of bronchoscopy in the diagnosis of airway disease. Journal of Thoracic Disease. 2016;**8**(12):3826-3837. DOI: 10.21037/jtd.2016.12.68

[7] Herth F, Ernst A, Schulz M, Becker H. Endobronchial ultrasound reliably differentiates between airway infiltration and compression by tumor. Chest. 2003;**123**:458-462. DOI: 10.1378/chest.123.2.458

[8] Herth F, Becker HD, Ernst A. Conventional vs endobronchial ultrasound-guided transbronchial needle aspiration: A randomized trial. Chest. 2004;**125**:322-325. DOI: 10.1378/chest.125.1.322

[9] Kurimoto N, Murayama M, Yoshioka S, Nishisaka T. Analysis of the internal structure of peripheral pulmonary lesions using endobronchial ultrasonography. Chest. 2002;**122**:1887-1894. DOI: 10.1378/chest.122.6.1887

[10] Yasufuku K, Nakajima T, Chiyo M, Sekine Y, Shibuya K, Fujisawa T. Endobronchial ultrasonography: Current status and future directions. Journal of Thoracic Oncology. 2007;**2**(10):970-979. DOI: 10.1097/JTO.0b013e318153fd8d

[11] Chandra S, Nehra M, Agarwal D, Mohan A. Diagnostics accuracy of endobronchial ultrasound-guided transbronchial needle biopsy in mediastinal lymphadenopathy: A systematic review and meta-analysis. Respiratory Care. 2012;**57**(3):384-391. DOI: 10.4187/respcare.01274

[12] Leong S, Ju H, Marshall H, et al. Electromagnetic navigation bronchoscopy: A descriptive analysis. Journal of Thoracic Disease. 2012;**4**(2):173-185. DOI: 10.3978/j.issn.2072-1439.2012.03.08

[13] Wang Memoli JS, Nietert PJ, Silvestri GA. Meta-analysis of guided bronchoscopy for the evaluation of the pulmonary nodule. Chest. 2012;**142**:385-393

[14] Harrison S, Port J. Electromagnetic navigational bronchoscopy. Seminars in Interventional Radiology. 2013;**30**:128-132

[15] Mahmoud N, Vashisht R, Sanghavi DK, Kalanjeri S. Bronchoscopy.

[Updated 2023 Jul 24]. In: StatPearls [Internet]. Treasure Island (FL): StatPearls Publishing; 2023. Available from: https://www.ncbi.nlm.nih.gov/books/NBK448152/

[16] Jacomelli M, Margotto SS, Demarzo SE, Scordamaglio PR, Cardoso PFG, Palomino ALM, et al. Early complications in flexible bronchoscopy at a university hospital. Jornal Brasileiro de Pneumologia. 2020;**46**(4). DOI: 10.36416/1806-3756/e20180125

[17] Du Rand IA, Blaikley J, Booton R, Chaudhuri N, Gupta V, Khalidet S. British Thoracic Society guideline for diagnostic flexible bronchoscopy in adults accredited by NICE. Thorax. 2013;**68**(1):1-44. DOI: 10.1136/thoraxjnl-2013-203618

[18] Pue CA, Pacht ER. Complications of fiberoptic bronchoscopy at a university hospital. Chest Journal. 1995;**107**(2): 430-432. DOI: 10.1378/chest.107.2.430

[19] Geraci G, Pisello F, Sciumè C, Li Volsi F, Romeo M, Modica G. Complication of flexible fiberoptic bronchoscopy: Literature review [Article in Italian]. Annali Italiani di Chirurgia. 2007;**78**(3):183-192

[20] Frazier WD, Pope TL Jr, Findley LJ. Pneumothorax following transbronchial biopsy Low diagnostic yield with routine chest roentgenograms. Chest Journal. 1990;**97**(3):539-540. DOI: 10.1378/chest.97.3.539

[21] Tukey MH, Wiener RS. Population-based estimates of transbronchial lung biopsy utilization and complications. Respiratory Medicine. 2012;**106**(11):1559-1565. DOI: 10.1016/j.rmed.2012.08.008

[22] Hernández Blasco L, Sánchez Hernández IM, Villena Garrido V, de Miguel PE, Nuñez Delgado M, Alfaro AJ. Safety of the transbronchial biopsy in outpatients. Chest Journal. 1991;**99**(3):562-565. DOI: 10.1378/chest.99.3.562

[23] Jin F, Mu D, Chu D, Fu E, Xie Y, Liu T. Severe complications of bronchoscopy. Respiration. 2008;**76**(4):429-433. DOI: 10.1159/000151656

[24] Carr IM, Koegelenberg CF, von Groote-Bidlingmaier F, Mowlana A, Silos K, Haverman T. Blood loss during flexible bronchoscopy a prospective observational study. Respiration. 2012;**84**(4):312-318. DOI: 10.1159/000339507

[25] Swanson KL, Edell ES. Tracheobronchial foreign bodies. Chest Surgery Clinics of North America. 2001;**11**(4):861-872

[26] Conlan AA, Hurwitz SS. Management of massive haemoptysis with the rigid bronchoscope and cold saline lavage. Thorax. 1980;**35**(12): 901-904. DOI: 10.1136/thx.35.12.901

[27] Colchen A, Fischler M. Bronchoscopies interventionnelles en urgence [Emergency interventional bronchoscopies]. Revue de pneumologie clinique. 2011;**67**(4):209-213. DOI: 10.1016/j.pneumo.2011.05.001

[28] Valipour A, Kreuzer A, Koller H, Koessler W, Burghuber OC. Bronchoscopy-guided topical hemostatic tamponade therapy for the management of life-threatening hemoptysis. Chest Journal. 2005;**127**(6):2113-2118. DOI: 10.1378/chest.127.6.2113

[29] Sakr L, Dutau H. Massive hemoptysis: An update on the role of bronchoscopy in diagnosis and management. Respiration. 2010;**80**(1):38-58. DOI: 10.1159/000274492

[30] Solomonov A, Fruchter O, Zuckerman T, Brenner B, Yigla M. Pulmonary hemorrhage: A novel mode of therapy. Respiratory Medicine. 2009;**103**(8):1196-1200. DOI: 10.1016/j.rmed.2009.02.004

[31] Casoni GL, Tomassetti S, Cavazza A, Colby TV, Dubini A, Ryu JH, et al. Transbronchial lung cryobiopsy in the diagnosis of fibrotic interstitial lung diseases. PLoS One. 2014;**9**(2):e86716. DOI: 10.1371/journal.pone.0086716

[32] Yarmus L, Akulian J, Gilbert C, Illei P, Shah P, Merlo C, et al. Cryoprobe transbronchial lung biopsy in patients after lung transplantation: a pilot safety study. Chest Journal. 2013;**143**(3):621-626. DOI: 10.1378/chest.12-2290

[33] Kropski JA, Pritchett JM, Mason WR, Sivarajan L, Gleaves LA, Johnson JE, et al. Bronchoscopic cryobiopsy for the diagnosis of diffuse parenchymal lung disease. PLoS One. 2013;**8**(11). DOI: 10.1371/journal.pone.0078674

[34] Grendelmeier P, Tamm M, Jahn K, Pflimlin E, Stolz D. Flexible bronchoscopy with moderate sedation in COPD: A case-control study. Journal of Chronic Obstructive Pulmonary Disease. 2017;**12**:177-187. DOI: 10.2147/COPD.S119575

[35] Bellinger CR, Khan I, Chatterjee AB, Haponik EF. Bronchoscopy safety in patients with chronic obstructive lung disease. Journal of Bronchology & Interventional Pulmonology. 2017;**24**(2):98-103. DOI: 10.1097/LBR.0000000000000333

[36] Li C, Zhu T, Ma D, Chen Y, Bo L. Complications and safety analysis of diagnostic bronchoscopy in COPD: A systematic review and meta-analysis. Expert Review of Respiratory Medicine. 2022;**16**(5):555-565. DOI: 10.1080/17476348.2022.2056023 Epub 2022 Apr 7

[37] Perotin JM, Dewolf M, Launois C, Dormoy V, Deslee G. Bronchoscopic management of asthma, COPD and emphysema. European Respiratory Review. 2021;**30**(159):200029. DOI: 10.1183/16000617.0029-2020

[38] Poggi C, Mantovani S, Pecoraro Y, Carillo C, Bassi M, D'Andrilli A, et al. Bronchoscopic treatment of emphysema: an update. Journal of Thoracic Disease. 2018;**10**(11):6274-6284. DOI: 10.21037/jtd.2018.10.43

[39] Global Initiative for Chronic Obstructive Lung Disease. Global Strategy for the Diagnosis, Management and Prevention of Chronic Obstructive Pulmonary Disease. 2020. Available from: https://goldcopd.org/gold-reports

[40] Klooster K, Ten Hacken NH, Slebos D. The lung volume reduction coil for the treatment of emphysema: A new therapy in development. Expert Review of Medical Devices. 2014;**11**:481-489. DOI: 10.1586/17434440.2014.929490

[41] Herth FJ, Eberhard R, Gompelmann D, et al. Bronchoscopic lung volume reduction with a dedicated coil: A clinical pilot study. Therapeutic Advances in Respiratory Disease. 2010;**4**:225-231. DOI: 10.1177/1753465810368553

[42] Gompelmann D, Shah PL, Valipour A, et al. Bronchoscopic thermal vapor ablation: Best practice recommendations from an expert panel on endoscopic lung volume reduction. Respiration. 2018;**95**:392-400

Chapter 5

Lung Deposition of Air Pollutants and Inhaled Drugs in Patients with Chronic Obstructive Pulmonary Disease (COPD) and Those on Non-Invasive Ventilation (NIV): Is It Still Challenging?

Radmila Dmitrovic and Isidora Simonovic

Abstract

Chronic Obstructive Pulmonary Disease (COPD) ranks among the leading causes of mortality worldwide, particularly in low- and middle-income nations. The primary risk factors for the development of COPD are tobacco smoking and the inhalation of pollutants from both indoor and outdoor sources. The exacerbation of COPD resulting from the mentioned factors significantly affects the patient's quality of life and is often associated with frequent hospitalizations and the potential need for mechanical ventilation. Regarding drug administration, the inhalation route is the most efficient way to deliver drugs directly to the lungs and target organs, while reducing systematic side effects. When evaluating the deposition of inhaled drugs in the lungs, the most frequently employed techniques are *in vivo*, scintigraphy, and functional respiratory imaging (FRI). Aside from bronchodilator therapy and corticosteroids, antibiotics, anti-inflammatory drugs, vaccines, and monoclonal antibodies are currently being studied for their potential benefits, particularly in patients receiving invasive or non-invasive mechanical ventilation.

Keywords: air pollution, lung deposition, NIV, drugs, techniques, FRI

1. Introduction

Based on recent data from the Global Initiative for Chronic Obstructive Lung Disease (GOLD), Chronic Obstructive Pulmonary Disease (COPD) ranks among the top three leading causes of death worldwide, particularly in low- and middle-income nations. The disease is characterized by respiratory symptoms, such as dyspnea, coughing, and exacerbation of symptoms in conditions that affect the airways (bronchitis/bronchiolitis) and/or the alveoli (emphysema). This leads to persistent and often progressive obstruction of the airways. The primary risk factors for the development of COPD are tobacco smoking and the inhalation of toxic particles from both indoor and outdoor sources [1]. This topic will focus on the subject of air pollution and its mechanisms of action, as well as the deposition of drugs in the lungs and the impact of this deposition on patients who are on mechanical ventilation.

2. Air pollutants and mechanism of action

According to data from the World Health Organization (WHO), ambient air pollution is responsible for 43% of cases of COPD, 29% of lung cancer cases, 25% of ischemic heart attack cases, and 24% of stroke-related deaths [2]. Air pollution refers to the presence of one or more substances in the air at concentrations or durations that exceed their normal levels, leading to harmful effects [3]. Certain air pollutants are of anthropogenic origin, arising from activities such as the combustion of fossil fuels. Others are a result of natural processes, such as particulate matter (PM), polycyclic aromatic hydrocarbons (PAHs), ozone, carbon dioxide (CO_2), and sulfur dioxide (SO2) [4]. **Figure 1** illustrates classification of air pollutants, outdoor and indoor pollutants [5]. Their mode of operation may vary. Ozone causes the oxidation of proteins and lipids in the fluid-lined compartments of the lungs, resulting in inflammation, increased permeability of the lungs, and the activation of pro-inflammatory cytokines, proteolytic enzymes, and reactive oxygen species (ROS). Ozone primarily affects the terminal bronchioles, the junction between the bronchioles and alveolar ducts, and the proximal alveolar regions. Lung inflammation caused by the inhalation of particulate matter is mediated by macrophages and epithelial cells. Alveolar macrophages have a significant impact on lung inflammation caused by particles, as they promote the production of interleukin 13 (IL-13) and interleukin 25 (IL-25) [6]. The mechanism of action of PM in COPD is illustrated in **Figure 2** [7].

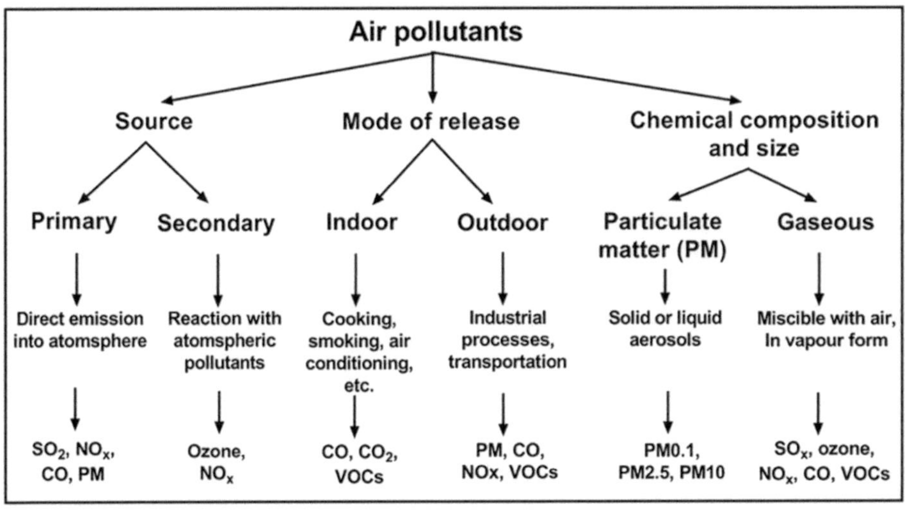

Figure 1.
Classification of air pollutants. CO-carbon monoxide, CO_2-carbon dioxide, NO_X- nitrogen oxides, PM- particle matter, PM0.1-particulate matter with particles of aerodynamic diameter < 0.1 μm, PM2.5- particulate matter with particles of aerodynamic diameter < 2.5 μm, PM10-particulate matter with particles of aerodynamic diameter < 10 μm, SO_X-sulfur oxide, SO_2-sulfur dioxide, VOC_s- volatile organic compounds.

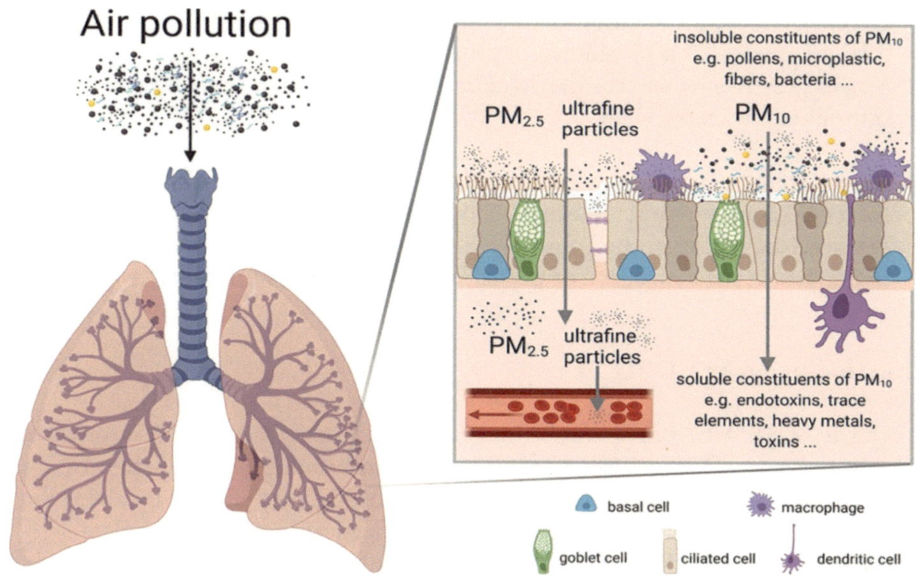

Figure 2.
Impact of PM2.5 and PM10 on COPD development.

Despite the anatomical positioning of the respiratory tract and its constant exposure to air pollutants in the atmosphere, many scientists continue to consider this topic to be controversial. A study involved over 400,000 patients who were exposed to various concentrations of air pollutants, including particulate matter (PM2.5 and PM10), nitrogen dioxide (NO_2), and nitrogen oxides (NOx). Their findings showed that individuals who had significant exposure to pollutants, an unfavorable lifestyle, and a high genetic predisposition were at a heightened risk of developing COPD [8].

3. Lung deposition—definition and main mechanism

The exacerbation of COPD resulting from the factors mentioned above significantly affects the quality of life for patients. This can lead to frequent hospitalizations and, in severe cases, the need for mechanical ventilation. A deposition is a process that determines what fraction of the inspired particles is caught in the lung and, thus fails to exit with expired air [9].

The primary mechanisms responsible for the transport and deposition of aerosols in the lungs are gravitational sedimentation, Brownian diffusion, and inertial impaction.

- Inertia is the resistance to changes in a moving object's speed and direction. It is a significant mechanism that applies to particles with diameters exceeding 2 μm. This mechanism necessitates a rapid flow and the deposition caused by inertial impaction will be influenced by the average flow. As per literature, inertia typically arises within the first 10 generations of the lungs due to high air velocity and turbulent airflow. As the size of particles decreases, the significance of inertia diminishes while the significance of diffusion increases.

- Gravitational sedimentation is the process by which particles settle due to the force of gravity. This phenomenon primarily occurs in narrow airways and alveolar cavities, where the particles have a short distance to travel before coming into contact with the walls.

- Brownian diffusion occurs due to random movements of particles resulting from their collisions with gas molecules. This phenomenon is especially prevalent in the acinar region of the lung, where air velocities are low. This mechanism dominates in the deposition of particles smaller than 0.5 μm [9–11].

4. Inhaled drugs in COPD

In terms of delivering drugs to the lungs and minimizing side effects throughout the body, the most efficient approach is through inhalation. Bronchodilatory therapy is frequently used in patients with COPD/asthma through dry powder inhalers (DPIs), soft-mist inhalers, nebulizers, and pressurized metered-dose inhalers (pMDIs). The therapeutic effects of inhaled medications are dependent upon various lung barriers, including humidity, mucociliary clearance, alveolar macrophages, and airway geometry. There is a positive correlation between the depth of deposition and the values of forced expiratory volume in the first second (FEV1). Patients with reduced FEV1 values will experience central deposition of the aerosolized drug in the lungs, unlike individuals with normal lung function. During an exacerbation, approximately 50% of the radio aerosol was eliminated from the lung within 97 minutes in patients with an FEV1 of 30–40%. In contrast, the clearance rate was less than 10% when the FEV1 was above 80%. A significant correlation was identified in cystic fibrosis (CF) [12, 13]. Scientific interest is focused on bronchodilator therapy, corticosteroids, antibiotics, anti-inflammatory drugs, vaccines, and monoclonal antibodies.

4.1 Inhaled antibiotics

Their administration aims to increase the local availability of drugs at the site of respiratory infections while minimizing systemic side effects. The most frequently administered antibiotics are aminoglycosides and fluoroquinolones due to their ability to attain the highest concentration in the respiratory system and exhibit the most potent antimicrobial activity. The administration of these drugs typically occurs through nebulization, inhalation, or aerosolization. Liposomal formulations of antibiotics and polymers represent the future of inhaled medications [14, 15]. The inhalable antibiotics that have been approved in Europe and the USA are listed in **Table 1** [23].

4.2 Anti-inflammatory drugs

Phosphodiesterase 4 (PDE4) inhibitors are frequently used. They do not directly affect systemic inflammation, but they can indirectly enhance the anti-inflammatory response, as shown by a decrease in exacerbations [24, 25]. The phosphatidylinositol 3-kinase (PI3K) plays a crucial role in COPD. PI3K activates various intracellular processes related to cell growth, proliferation, metabolism, and survival by facilitating the synthesis of phosphatidylinositol-3,4,5-triphosphate (PIP3). The most crucial component is nemiralisib, which, when used initially, has been found to enhance lung

	Antibiotic	Agency	Approved indications	References
1	Aztreonam inhalation solution (Cayston®)	EMA/ FDA	To suppress chronic pulmonary infections due to *Pseudomonas aeruginosa* in patients with CF, 6 years of age and FEV_1 25–75% predicted (EU)	CAYSTON® summary of product characteristics [16]
			To improve respiratory symptoms in CF patients with *P. aeruginosa*, 7 years of age and with FEV_1 25–75% predicted (US)	CAYSTON® prescribing information [17]
			Treatment schedule is 28-days-on drug alternating with 28-days-off drug	
2	Colistimethate sodium inhalation solution (Colistin)	EMA	Colistin: For management of chronic infections due to *P. aeruginosa* in patients with CF, adults and children	Promixin® summary of product characteristics [18]
	Colistimethate sodium inhalation powder (Colobreathe®)		Colobreathe®: For management of chronic infections due to *P. aeruginosa* in patients with CF aged ≥6 years	Colobreathe® summary of product characteristics [19]
			Treatment schedule is a continuous regimen	
3	Levofloxacin nebulizer solution (QUINSAIR®)	EMA/ FDA	For management of chronic pulmonary infections due to *P. aeruginosa* in adult patients with CF	Quinsair® summary of product characteristics [20]
			Treatment schedule is 28-days-on drug alternating with 28-days-off drug	
4	Tobramycin inhalation solution (TOBI®)	EMA/ FDA	TOBI®: For management of CF patients with *P. aeruginosa*, 6 years of age and with FEV_1 25–75% predicted	TOBI® prescribing information [21]
			TOBI® Podhaler™: For management of CF patients with *P. aeruginosa*, 6 years of age and with FEV_1 25–80% predicted (US) or 25–75% predicted (EU)	TOBI® Podhaler™ prescribing information [22]
	Tobramycin inhalation powder (TOBI® Podhaler™)			
			Treatment schedule is 28-days-on drug alternating with 28-days-off drug	

CF, cystic fibrosis; EMA, European Medicines Agency; EU, European Union; FDA, US Food and Drug Administration; FEV_1, forced expiratory volume in 1 second; US, United States.

Table 1.
Inhaled antibiotics in Europe and USA.

function for a duration of 3 months by mitigation [26]. The p38 mitogen-activated protein kinases (MAPK) regulate the apoptosis of macrophages and neutrophils, as well as induce the release of cytokines and chemokines from these cells, including interleukin 1β (IL-1β), tumor necrosis factor-α (TNF-α), interleukin 8 (IL-8), interleukin 17A (IL-17A), and interleukin 17F (IL-17F). This collective action facilitates the recruitment and activation of neutrophils. The significance of blocking p38 MAPKs in COPD is demonstrated by all of these effects [27].

4.3 Inhaled vaccines

The administration of vaccines through inhalation allows for targeting all areas of the respiratory system and has the potential to serve as a needle-free alternative. The vaccine can be administered directly, stimulating a localized immune response aided by immunoglobulin A (IgA) antibodies. It can also be administered to the respiratory mucosa, inducing systematic immunoglobulin G (IgG)-mediated and cell-mediated responses. Vaccines must possess specific properties to be administered via inhalation:

a. Due to the insufficient ability to induce an immune response when used alone, the antigen must be presented in a particulate form and always be administered together with an adjuvant that is effective in stimulating the mucosal immune system.

b. The formulation must have the ability to be administered through an appropriate device.

Traditionally, vaccines have been produced in liquid and powder forms. However, in recent years, researchers have developed dried vaccines that can maintain their *in vivo* efficacy [22, 28].

4.4 Monoclonal antibodies (mAbs)

Administering monoclonal antibodies (mAbs) via inhalation is currently a complex and appealing practice in the field of medicine. Delivering mAbs in this manner is characterized by a quick onset of action, enhanced effectiveness at lower doses, minimal systematic exposure, and reduced likelihood of negative drug reactions. The drug's mechanism of action involves specifically targeting the airways and the tissue site of cytokine expression. The lungs possess a large surface area, with airway epithelium that is extremely thin and well vascularized. As a result, absorption occurs quickly and the onset of action is rapid. The most frequently mentioned mAbs are pharmacokinetics (PK) and pharmacodinamics (PD) of CSJ117 was evaluated in one study. A randomized, placebo-controlled, participant- and investigator-blinded study was conducted at multiple centers to evaluate the impact of CSJ117 on individuals with COPD. The main result analyzed was the difference in the Evaluating Respiratory Symptoms (E-RS) score compared to the baseline value. The study was concluded in 2022, and there are currently no available results. In addition, it is necessary to conduct randomized control trials (RCTs) to evaluate the possible effectiveness of these drugs in treating COPD [16].

5. Scintigraphy and functional respiratory imaging (FRI)

The effectiveness of delivering drugs to the lungs is determined by a combination of several factors: the physicochemical characteristics of the drug, the drug's formulation, the type of inhalation device used (such as pressurized metered-dose inhalers, dry powder inhalers, nebulizers, or soft-mist inhalers), as well as factors related to the patient and the disease (such as breathing pattern and airway constriction). Except for bronchoalveolar lavage and tissue biopsies, which have inherent limitations, accurately measuring drug concentrations in the lung tissue of humans is an arduous task. Non-invasive nuclear medicine imaging techniques have significant potential. The imaging techniques used for this purpose are planar gamma scintigraphy, single-photon emission computed tomography (SPECT), and positron emission tomography (PET). Nuclear medicine imaging techniques enable the dynamic measurement of radiolabeled molecule concentrations in the lungs, known as radiotracers. There are three ways in which these imaging techniques can be utilized. The first method involves the process of radiolabeling a component of the drug formulation, such as solid particles or solvent, with the assumption that this component will exhibit similar behavior to the drug present in the formulation. This approach is commonly utilized in lung deposition studies. The second method involves the process of radiolabeling the drug molecule directly. The said process is technically more demanding due to the requirement of devising a radiolabeling strategy for the desired medication and subsequently incorporating the radiolabeled drug into the inhalation device. It provides a significant benefit, such as the ability to evaluate the drug's retention in the lungs over time as well as clearance processes from the lungs. The third approach utilizes an imaging biomarker to assess the impact of the inhaled drug, specifically by measuring target receptor occupancy. Although this method will yield important information regarding the effectiveness of delivering drugs to the lungs, it depends on understanding the specific drug target and having a radiotracer available to measure the binding of the inhaled drug to this target (**Figure 3**) [17].

Functional respiratory imaging (FRI) involves the application of non-invasive, three-dimensional lung models created from high-resolution computed tomography scans (HRCT). These models are then analyzed using computational fluid dynamics

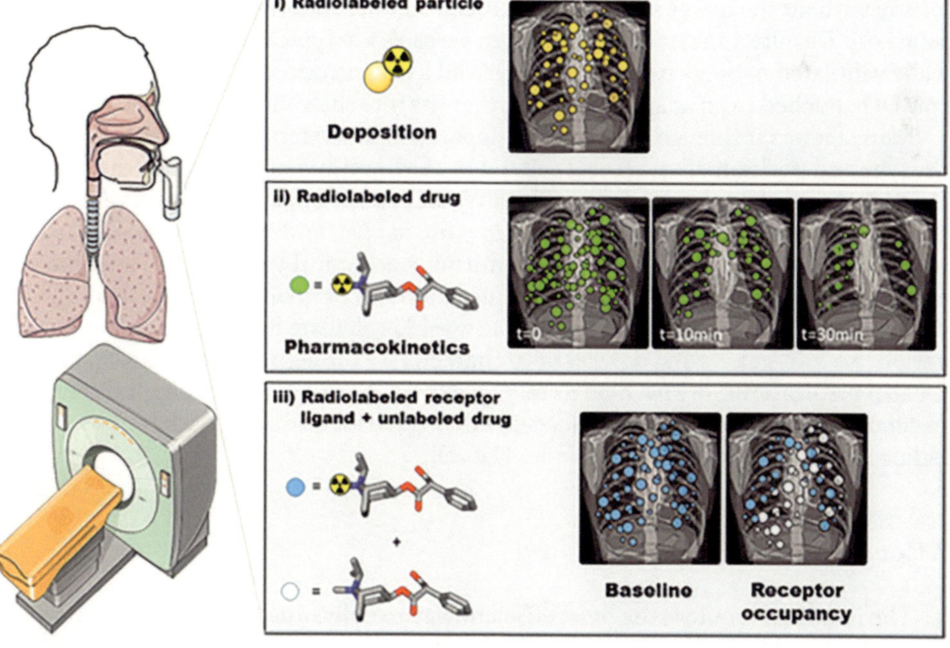

Figure 3.
Illustration of the three access of nuclear medicine imaging methods in lung deposition: (I) planar gamma scintigraphy with radiolabeled inhalation formulations to assess initial pulmonary drug deposition, (II) PET imaging studies with radiolabeled drugs to assess their intrapulmonary pharmacokinetics and (III) receptor occupancy studies to quantify the pharmacodynamic effect of an inhaled drug.

(CFD). Compared to scintigraphy, FRI enables the modeling of patient-specific deposition in peripheral airways without requiring patient recruitment. This technique is based on three phases:

1. Medical imaging: The process commences by obtaining a low-dose, high-resolution computed tomography (HRCT) scan of the patient.

2. Imaging processing: Measurements are conducted on the segmented three-dimensional geometries obtained from these scans.

3. Flow simulation: CFD is used to quantify airflow and exposure to inhaled particles [18].

In one study, *Pseudomonas aeruginosa* was treated with inhaled levofloxacin in CF patients. The antibiotic's lung deposition was predicted using FRI. The FRI demonstrated substantial intrathoracic deposition of levofloxacin, with a preference for distribution in the lower lung lobes. The ratio of central to peripheral deposition (C/P) was influenced by the decline in FEV1. In addition, structural distinctions between patients with mild and moderate CF were identified by the three-dimensional rendering of CF airways [19].

6. Inhaled drugs and non-invasive ventilation (NIV)

Non-invasive ventilation (NIV) is defined as positive pressure ventilation in the airway without the use of an invasive artificial airway, endotracheal, or tracheostomy tube [20]. Despite appearances, medicated aerosols are typically delivered to mechanically ventilated patients using a nebulizer and a pressurized metered-dose inhaler (pMDI) attached to an adapter or spacer that fits into the ventilated circuit.

Many factors influence inhaled drug deposition in the lungs during NIV, including the type and position of an aerosol generator, the humidity of the circuit, the characteristics of aerosolized particles, gas density, the type of patient interface, ventilator parameters, and patient-related factors. *In vitro, in vivo*, and *ex vivo* models are used to study aerosol delivery and deposition during mechanical ventilation. These models are dependent on the technique used to quantitatively or qualitatively measure the deposited aerosol. *In vitro* models could be used to calculate total emitted doses from various aerosol-generating devices or to characterize the aerodynamics of deposited inhaled medications. *In vivo* models rely on extracting drugs from biological samples to determine concentration and bioavailability (pharmacokinetic model) or on radioactive aerosol imaging techniques [21, 29].

7. Conclusion

The inhalation route is the most efficient way to deliver drugs directly to the lungs and target organs, while reducing systematic side effects, especially in those patients on NIV. This way of drug application was recognized a couple of decades ago but it is still unknown to physicians. It is necessary to educate physicians about groups of drugs that are applied in this way, the way of their application, and the methods by which the concentration of the inhaled drug is monitored.

DOI: http://dx.doi.org/10.5772/intechopen.1004263

Author details

Radmila Dmitrovic[1]* and Isidora Simonovic[2]

1 Department of Pulmonology, Clinical Hospital Center "Zemun", Belgrade, Serbia

2 Emergency Department, Clinical Hospital Center "Zemun", Belgrade, Serbia

*Address all correspondence to: radadmitrovic94@gmail.com

References

[1] Global strategies for the diagnosis, management and prevention of chronic obstructive pulmonary disease (2023 Report). Available from: https://goldcopd.org/2023-gold-report-2/

[2] World Health Organization. Ambient Air Pollution. World Health Organization; 2022. Available from: https://www.who.int/data/gho/data/themes/topics/indicatorgroups/indicator-group-details/GHO/ambient-air-pollution

[3] Senfield JH, Pandis S. Atmospheric Chemistry and Physics. 2nd ed. Hoboken (NJ): John Wiley; 2006

[4] IARC Working Group on the Evaluation of Carcinogenic Risks to Humans. Outdoor Air Pollution. Lyon (FR): International Agency for Research on Cancer; 2016. Available from: https://www.ncbi.hlm.nih.gov/books/NBK368034

[5] Kadam V. Multifunctional air filtration for respiratory protection using electrospun nanofibre membrane [thesis]. Australia: RMIT University; 2018

[6] Lee YG, Lee PH, Choi SM, An MH, Jang AS. Effects of air pollutants on airway disease. International Journal of Environmental Research and Public Health. 2021;**18**(18):9905

[7] Misiukiewicz-Stepien P et al. Biological effect of PM10 on airway epithelium-focus on obstructive lung disease. Clinical Immunology. 2021;**227**:108754

[8] Wang L, Xie J, Hu Y, Tian Y. Air pollution and risk of chronic obstructed pulmonary disease: The modifying effect of genetic susceptibility and life style. eBioMedicine. 2022;**79**:103994

[9] National Research Council (US). Panel on Dosimetric Assumptions Affecting the Application of Radon Risk Estimates. Comparative Dosimetry of Radon in Mines and Homes. Washington (DC): National Academies Press (US); 1991. Available from: https://www.ncbi.nlm.nih.gov/books/NBK234222/

[10] Darquenne C. Aerosol deposition in health and disease. Journal of Aerosol Medicine and Pulmonary Drug Delivery. 2012;**25**(3):140-147

[11] Darquenne C, Prisk KG. Aerosol deposition in the human respiratory tract breathing air and 80:20 Heliox. Journal of Aerosol Medicine. 2004;**17**(3):278-285

[12] Labris NR, Dolovich MB. Pulmonary drug delivery. Part I: Physiological factors affecting therapeutic effectiveness of aerosolized medications. British Journal of Clinical Pharmacology. 2003;**56**(6):588-599

[13] Cazzola M, Ora J, Calzetta L, Rogliani P, Matera MG. The future of inhalation therapy in chronic obstructive pulmonary disease. Current Research in Pharmacology and Drug Discovery. 2022;**3**:100092

[14] Restrepo MI, Keyt H, Reyes LF. Aerosolized antibiotics. Respiratory Care. 2015;**60**(16):762-761

[15] Carrillo DR, Martínez-García MA, Barreiro E, Huguet ET, Costa Sola R, García-Clemente MM, et al. Effectiveness and safety of inhaled antibiotics in patients with chronic obstructive pulmonary disease. A multicentre observational study. Archivos de Bronconeumología. 2022;**58**(1):11-21

[16] Laitano R, Calzetta L, Cavali F, Cazzola M, Rogliani P. Delivering

monoclonal antibodies via inhalation: A systematic review of clinical trials in asthma and COPD. Expert Opinion on Drug Delivery. 2023;**20**(8):1041-1054

[17] Mairinger S, Hernández-Lozano I, Zeintliger M, Erhardt C, Langer O. Nuclear medicine imaging methods as novel tools in the assessment of pulmonary drug disposition. Expert Opinion on Drug Delivery. 2022;**19**(12):1561-1575

[18] Usmani OS, Mignot B, Kendall I, Maria R, Cocconi D, Georges G, et al. Predicting lung deposition of extrafine inhaled corticosteroid-containing fixed combinations in patients with chronic obstructive pulmonary disease using functional respiratory imaging: An in silico study. Journal of Aerosol Medicine and Pulmonary Drug Delivery. 2021;**34**(3):204-211

[19] Schwarz C, Procaccianti C, Mignot B, Sadafi H, Schwenck N, Murgia X, et al. Deposition of inhaled levofloxacin in cystic fibrosis lungs assessed by functional respiratory imaging. Pharmaceutics. 2021;**13**(12):2051

[20] Lazovic B, Dmitrovic R, Simonovic I, Esquinas AM. Assessment of noninvasive ventilation (NIV) effectiveness in the COVID19 infection: A clinical review. Med Data. 2021;**13**:163-165

[21] Saeed H, Harb HS, Madney Y, Abdelrahim MEA. Aerosol delivery via noninvasive ventilation: Role of models and bioanalysis. Annals of Translational Medicine. 2021;**9**(7):589

[22] Kaur SS. Pulmonary drug delivery system: Newer patents. Pharmaceutical Patent Analyst. 2017;**6**(5):225-244

[23] Hamed K, Debonnet L. Tobramycin inhalation powder for the treatment of pulmonary *Pseudomonas aeruginosa* infection in patients with cystic fibrosis: A review based on clinical evidence. Therapeutic Advances in Respiratory Disease. 2017;**11**(5):193-209

[24] Phillips EJ. Inhaled phosphodiesterase 4 (PDE4) inhibitors for inflammatory respiratory disease. Frontiers in Pharmacology. 2020;**11**:259

[25] Singh D, Emirova A, Francisco C, Santoro D, Govoni M, Nandeuil MA. Efficacy and safety of CHF6001, a novel inhaled PDE4 inhibitor in COPD: The PIONEER study. Respiratory Research. 2020;**21**:246

[26] Cazzola M, Page CP, Calzetta L, Matera MG. Emerging anti-inflammatory strategies for COPD. The European Respiratory Journal. 2012;**40**(3):724-741

[27] Limón-Martínez A, Joaquin M, Caballero M, Posas F, Nadal E. The p38 pathway: From biology to cancer therapy. International Journal of Molecular Sciences. 2020;**21**(6):1913

[28] Heida R, Hinrichs WLJ, Frijlink HW. Inhaled vaccine delivery in the combat against respiratory viruses: A 2021 overview of recent developments and implications for COVID-19. Expert Review of Vaccines. 2022;**21**(7):957-974

[29] Dhand R, Guntur VP. How best to deliver aerosol medication to mechanically ventilated patients. Clinics in Chest Medicine. 2008;**29**(2):277-296

Chapter 6

Lung Transplantation as a Treatment Strategy for Pulmonary Emphysema

Alina Ligia Cornea, Seamus Linnane, Peter Riddell, Diana Parau and Alexandru Mihai Cornea

Abstract

The role of lung transplantation is to provide survival and quality of life benefits to patients with advanced lung disease. In this chapter, focusing on chronic obstructive pulmonary disease (COPD), we provide a comprehensive discussion of key aspects involved in the assessment of recipient suitability for transplantation. We discuss key issues such as timing of referral, donor evaluation, and organ allocation. We provide a detailed evaluation of the technical aspects of transplant surgery, evaluating the relative merits of both single and bilateral lung transplantation. In addition, we highlight how the transplant field is addressing donor shortfall, with expansion of acceptable donor criteria and the use of *ex vivo* lung perfusion to improve donor evaluation. Finally, we examine post-operative morbidity and mortality, discussing both early and late surgical complications and the adverse effects of long-term immunosuppression.

Keywords: lung transplantation, chronic obstructive pulmonary disease, donation after circulatory death, single lung transplantation, double lung transplantation, early and late outcomes

1. Introduction

Lung transplantation (LTx) is a surgical intervention that aims to provide survival and quality of life (QoL) benefits to patients with advanced lung disease. However, this intervention is associated with significant peri-operative and long-term adverse risks. Identifying suitable candidates therefore requires a detailed evaluation of recipient risk factors by a multi-disciplinary team.

Chronic obstructive pulmonary disease (COPD) is one of the most frequent indications for LTx, accounting for approximately one-third of cases worldwide [1]. However, despite the high symptom burden as lung function declines, identifying patients who will achieve a survival benefit from LTx is not always straightforward. Multimodal assessment of lung function, exercise tolerance, and symptom burden (e.g. the BODE index) provides a good reference point for referral for transplant. However, additional factors that increase mortality risk from COPD, such as the development of pulmonary hypertension or chronic hypercapnia may influence listing decisions.

As an alternative to LTx, either as a temporizing intervention or for patients unsuitable for LTx, lung volume reduction techniques (surgical or bronchoscopic) may also be considered. However, these techniques also require specific eligibility criteria to be met, such as upper lobe predominant disease, so are not suitable for all patients. In selected cohorts, however, lung volume reduction can result in significant improvement in quality of life and exercise levels.

2. Transplant as a therapeutic option for emphysema in COPD patients

2.1 COPD as a progressive condition

The pathogenesis of COPD is characterized by chronic airway inflammation, resulting in fixed airflow limitation and alveolar wall destruction. Prolonged exposure to cigarette smoke is the key risk factor [2], but environmental exposures (vapors, dust, and workplace pollutants) have also been associated with the pathogenesis of this condition. Genetic risk factors, in particular alpha-1 antitrypsin (A1AT) deficiency, are also of importance [3]. Smoking also has the potential to affect other comorbidities that progress in tandem with COPD and can negatively impact functional status, survival, and fitness for transplant surgery.

2.2 Epidemiology of COPD

The natural history of COPD is characterized by increasing morbidity over time, which leads to increasing disability, respiratory failure, and eventually death. Transplantation therefore has the potential to confer quality of life and survival benefits to this cohort of patients. However, due to the risks involved, it is typically pursued only after all other treatment modalities have been exhausted.

COPD is highly prevalent. The WHO recognizes this condition as the third highest cause of mortality worldwide [4]. Given such a large denominator, it is apparent that only a very small percentage of COPD patients benefit from transplantation. The implementation of lung transplants is therefore highly specialized and is reserved for highly selected cases, where survival and QoL benefits are likely to be achieved. It is best considered within the setting of a specialist tertiary or quaternary center that operates in a hub-and-spoke service model to ensure equitable and geographically diverse access within a unified healthcare system.

2.3 Subtypes of COPD

A1AT deficiency is caused by a single gene abnormality, prevalent in certain populations [5]. A1AT inhibits elastase that when activated unopposed causes enzymatic destruction of host tissue. An imbalance in protease:anti-protease activity due to the functional reduction or absence of A1AT predisposing to development lung (COPD and bronchiectasis) and liver disease [6]. These observations were for many years the foundation of the elastase/anti-elastase pathogenesis hypothesis of COPD [7]. Diagnosis and family screening are crucial to identify patients with early or progressive disease [8]. Smoking cessation or, more importantly, avoidance is therefore the most significant treatment intervention [9].

Patients with A1AT deficiency who present with emphysema tend to do so at a younger age with fewer comorbidities and less functional impairment. Transplant registries tend to overrepresent A1AT deficiency among their emphysema cohorts due to these differences in clinical presentation, comorbid burden, and age [10]. Patients with A1AT deficiency as the defining reason for enrollment in a lung transplant program tend to have better outcomes [11]. For patients with A1AT deficiency who have developed concomitant lung and liver disease, multi-organ transplant may be necessary, but requires careful co-management in a center of excellence, to optimize the timing of transplantation and the quality of patient [12].

2.4 Survival in COPD

Predicting survival in COPD can be challenging, as disease progression does not follow a linear trend [13]. The BODE index is a tool that assists clinics with disease prognostication [14]. This simple clinical index considers airway obstruction measured by spirometry, physical features such as body mass index, exercise capacity measured using a six-minute walk test, and symptom score measured using the modified Medical Research Council dyspnoea scale. However, as the score was not originally developed to assess surgical patients, it may overestimate mortality risk in younger patients [15]. Modification using data from transplant registries may refine this index in surgical candidates in the future.

2.5 Comorbidities in COPD

COPD may be considered a multisystem disease not just limited to the lung. Smoking-related diseases of other organs can impede progression to transplantation. For example, atherosclerotic disease prevalence increases with cigarette smoking and advancing age. Atherosclerosis is frequent in those with emphysema, and studies have identified emphysema as an independent risk factor for coronary artery disease with a bi-directional relationship [16].

Coronary artery disease is frequently concordant with sclerosis of other vascular beds such as those of the cerebral circulation. As such, the identification and optimization of coronary artery and established vascular disease are prerequisites for patient selection and acceptance into a transplant program.

A host of other comorbidities are associated with COPD including metabolic syndrome, osteoporosis, sarcopenia, and malignancy [17]. These require identification and management and can have a variable impact on selection and management of lung transplant. They also increase the overall recipient risk profile as many of the symptoms are exacerbated by post-transplant immunosuppression. The complex permutations, combinations, and interplay of disparate pathophysiological processes create a heterogeneous patient population underscoring the importance of comprehensive and multi-disciplinary management.

2.6 Surgical management of COPD

The choice of the transplant procedure depends on various factors, including whether it involves a single lung, bilateral lung, or multi-organ transplant [18]. Multi-organ transplants may occur in tandem or sequentially, depending on clinical need. Lung transplant is not the only potential surgical intervention for patients with COPD; lung volume reduction surgery and other interventional therapies, such as endobronchial coils and valves, also have a role to play [19]. These enhanced surgical techniques may be part of or ancillary to a lung transplant program. Therefore, a patient may be referred for general surgical consideration, with lung transplant being one option among several considered by the thoracic transplant team.

In certain circumstances, lung transplant may follow other surgical approaches that act as a temporary measure or a bridge to transplant. Transplant surgery may be deferred, while patient care and performance status are optimized. The management of patients who have undergone prior surgical procedures may require additional consideration by the transplant team [20].

2.7 Prognosis and transplant

Patient selection for lung transplantation is based on a detailed assessment of a potential candidate's individual risk profile. This assessment should involve a multidisciplinary team of sub-specialty experts that includes transplant anaesthesiology, surgery, critical care, and pulmonology. The overriding principle of this decision-making process is to decide whether lung transplantation (assuming adequate allograft function) will be associated will survival and QoL benefits that are greater than medical management alone (i.e. no transplant).

This paradigm dictates that the morbidity and mortality associated with the intervention should be offset by the expected survival gain from treatment using a balanced risk-benefit assessment approach [21]. Conversely, the prognosis of the patient being selected for surgery should be significantly grave to achieve a survival advantage offered by the procedure. Paradoxically a poor short-term prognosis is often correlated with worsening performance status, making patients less suitable for surgery than their longer-lived counterparts.

2.8 Principles of patient selection

Given the scarcity of lung transplant as a life-saving treatment option, fairness and equity of access are particularly important and subject to justifiable societal scrutiny. An international consortium of the International Society for Heart and Lung Transplantation (ISHLT) provides consensus documents to facilitate the selection of patients by presenting appropriate, clinically based criteria. The current document [22], suggests that adults with chronic end-stage lung disease should have a two-year survival of less than 50 percent in the absence of transplant and a greater than 80 percent expected survival at 5 years, assuming adequate graft function post-treatment. Absolute contraindications have been emphasized in earlier documents [23] while relative contraindications may be tackled in centers with expertise in dealing with those specific contraindications.

2.9 Relative contraindications for lung transplantation

Advancing recipient age at the time of lung transplantation has been reported to adversely impact five-year survival [24]. Arbitrarily age-related cut-offs are avoided by most transplant programs, focusing instead on a potential recipient's overall fitness — biological rather than chronological age — for transplant. However, in view of age-related-adverse risk, the 2021 ISHLT consensus statement describes an age between 65 and 70 years to be associated with unfavorable short and/or long-term outcomes. Furthermore, an age greater than 70 years at transplant is associated with substantially increased adverse risk [25].

Obesity also increases short-term and long-term post-operative complications and should be optimized as part of a pre-operative management algorithm [26]. Low body mass index also confers a similar risk. Nicotine dependence, identified through screening, requires explicit medical advice regarding abstinence. Tobacco abstinence can be confirmed using either cotinine or exhaled carbon monoxide measurement as part of a smoking cessation adherence program. Vaping of nicotine salts or products is harder to define and detect though also a concern [27]. A significant period of abstinence before surgery is a usual component of most programs. Despite the importance of this issue, ongoing tobacco abuse is surprisingly prevalent [28], with disappointing rates of cessation given the nature of the LT intervention.

2.10 Disease-specific triggers for transplant

A BODE score of greater than five is considered sufficient to initiate a referral for transplant assessment. Other factors to consider include the exacerbation phenotype of the patient, as frequent exacerbators have poor survival. More than one exacerbation per year represents a significant increase in short-term survival risk. Dynamic deterioration, such as an increasing BODE score by a unit of one in the previous 12 months, encourages referral. The ISHLT consensus recommends admission to a lung transplant waiting list for those with a BODE score in the range of 7–10, with an FEV-1 less than 20% of predicted and evidence of moderate rehabilitation potential [29]. Other factors associated with increased mortality risk, such as the development of pulmonary hypertension or hypercapnia, may also prompt transplant listing.

3. Recipient selection and listing criteria for LT for COPD

Performing a lung transplant for COPD presents significant challenges, with a path marked by numerous potential pitfalls and complexities. Determining the optimal timing for transplantation in these cases poses a challenge due to the prolonged stability observed in patients with consistent oxygen requirements. This timeframe is often referred to as the "transplant window", representing the ideal period for offering an LT with the highest chance of success [30].

3.1 Referral for LT assessment

A patient with COPD is typically referred for LT when medical interventions have been exhausted and a decline in general health status has occurred. The 2021 ISHLT consensus statement on candidate selection, recommends referral for transplant assessment when the following criteria are met:

1. A BODE score of 5–6, in addition to one of the following:

    a. Frequent acute exacerbations

    b. Increase in BODE score > 1 point over 24 months

    c. FEV1 20–25% predicted

2. Clinical deterioration despite maximal medical management

3. Quality of life that the patient considers to be unacceptably poor

3.2 Listing for LT

Patients typically meet specific listing criteria for COPD, characterized by advanced disease, usually at Global Initiative for Chronic Obstructive Lung Disease (GOLD) stage IV [30].

In an otherwise suitable lung transplant candidate, achieving a BODE score of 7–10, associated with increased mortality risk, is recommended as the cut-off for transplant listing. Other factors, also associated with mortality risks, such as the presence of moderate-to-severe pulmonary hypertension, an FEV1, 20% predicted, a history of severe acute exacerbations, or the presence of chronic hypercapnia may also prompt listing, irrespective of BODE score [22].

4. Contraindications for LT

Certain contraindications for LT are considered absolute, (see **Table 1**) such as the presence of high-grade malignancy (<5 years), acute medical instability due to acute myocardial ischemia, irreversible multi organ failure, septic shock, severe coagulopathy, active substance abuse (alcohol, nicotine, marijuana, etc.), inadequate social support or nonadherence to medical therapy. Other risk factors are determinants for an increased chance of complications or unfavorable posttransplant outcome [22].

Absolute contraindications	**Risk factors with high or substantially increased risk**	**Risk factors with unfavorable implications of posttransplant outcome**
Candidates with these conditions are considered too high-risk to achieve successful outcomes post lung transplantation	Candidates with these conditions maybe considered in centers with expertise specific to the condition	While acceptable for lung transplant programs to consider patients with these risk factors, multiple risk factors together may increase the risk of adverse post-lung transplant outcomes
Factor or condition that significantly increases the risk of an adverse outcome post-transplant is most likely harmful for a recipient.	We may not have data to support transplanting patients with these risk factors or there is substantially increased risk based upon the currently available data, and further research is needed to better inform future recommendations.	
Most lung transplant programs should not transplant patients with these risk factors except under very exceptional or extenuating circumstances.	When more than one of these risk factors is present, they are thought to be possibly multiplicative in terms of increasing risk of adverse outcomes. Modifiable conditions should be optimized when possible.	

Absolute contraindications	Risk factors with high or substantially increased risk	Risk factors with unfavorable implications of posttransplant outcome
1. Lack of patient willingness or acceptance of Tx 2. Malignancy with high-risk of recurrence or death 3. Glomerular filtration<40 mL/min/1.73 m^2, unless considered for multi-organ Tx 4. Acute coronary artery syndrome or myocardial infarction within 30 days 5. Stroke within 30 days 6. Liver cirrhosis with portal hypertension or synthetic dysfunction unless considered for multi-organ Tx 7. Other conditions (Acute liver failure, Septic shock, active tuberculosis, etc.)	1. Age over 70 years 2. Severe coronary artery disease requires coronary artery bypass grafting 3. Reduced left ventricular ejection fraction <40% 4. Sugnificant cerebrovascular disease 5. Severe esophageal dysmotility 6. Untreatable hematologic disorders including bleeding diathesis, thrombophilia, or severe bone marrow dysfunction. Other factors as BMI > than or equal to 45 Kg/m^2, Psychiatric conditions, Mycobacterium infections, etc.)	1. Age 65–70 years 2. Glomerular filtration rate 40–60 mL/min/1.73 m^2 3. Mild to moderate coronary artery disease 4. Severe coronary artery disease that can be revascularized via percutaneous coronary intervention prior to transplant 5. Patient with prior coronary artery bypass grafting 6. Reduced left ejection fraction 40–50% 7. Other factors (peripheral vascular disease, connective tissue disorders, severe gastroesophageal reflux disease, etc.)

Table 1.
Risk factors for poor posttransplant outcomes.

5. Donor lung evaluation

Currently, there is a shortage of available lung donors, resulting in a higher number of patients on waiting lists compared to the number of donors that are suitable for LT. However, there is a wide variation in donor acceptance rates across the world [31]. This may be associated with variability in healthcare models, prioritization of donor management in ICUs, and access to advanced assessment techniques, such as EVLP.

6. Ideal donor selection

Ideal donor selection criteria are depicted in **Table 2**. The prevailing donor criteria are seldom met in contemporary settings, with only 15–25% of lung donors meeting these ideal criteria [33].

7. Extended criteria donors (ECD)

Consequently, ECDs have been devised to address these limitations. Commonly encountered extended donor lung criteria encompass anomalies in chest X-rays, a documented history of smoking, and marginal gas exchange levels. Lungs from

Ideal Donor selection criteria
Age < 55 years
No history of pulmonary disease
Normal serial chest radiograph
Normal gas exchange
Normal bronchoscopy
Size matching
Negative serologic screening for hepatitis B, and C and HIV
Recipient matching for ABO blood group

Table 2.
Ideal donor selection criteria [32].

donors more than 55 years old are now accepted for donation regularly [22]. Donors aged 60–70 are still considered eligible for donation despite evidence indicating that older ages have a higher 10-year mortality rate. The ECD also includes donors after pulmonary embolism or history of cancer or hypoxia-exposed lungs (less than 300 mm Hg which are now accepted for donation [33]. The use of lungs from donors with hepatitis B or C has been reported to be safe on both early and late treatment after lung transplantation [34]. The incorporation of the extended criteria has the potential to augment the donor pool by 50% [35].

In recent years, two additional approaches have emerged to address donor shortage; donation after cardiac death (DCD) and *ex vivo* lung perfusion (EVLP). EVLP, specifically serves as a technique for the functional assessment of lungs, determining their suitability for transplantation by evaluating their viability and usability [35].

The ideal lung donor selection criteria are summarized in **Table 2** [32].

7.1 Brain-death heart-beating donors (DBD)

The predominant source of lung donations from transplantation comes from brain-dead heart-beating donors, largely due to widespread acceptance of brain death legislation across numerous countries. Japan stands out as an exception where the lack of legislation on DBD for many years spurred the development of living donor lung donations to boost the availability of lungs for transplant surgeries [36].

The assessment of donor lungs commences upon arrival at the donor hospital and involves multiple procedures. All pertinent information, including the donor's medical history, cause of death, hospitalization detailed testing including ECGs, echocardiograms, chest X-rays, CT scans of the chest, ventilation support, medications administered (such as inotropes, diuretics, steroids), central venous pressures, arterial gas measurements, urine output, and pulmonary artery pressure, are carefully considered [36]. A checklist for donors can be employed to ensure that no details are overlooked see **Table 3** [37].

7.1.1 Intraoperative assessment of the donor

The evaluation process begins with bronchoscopy aimed at examining the bronchial anatomy for abnormalities, presence of secretions, foreign bodies, or other anomalies. Any secretions are cleared, and samples are collected for microbiological analysis through

Upon Arrival at the Procurement Center
Consent for donation
Verification of brain death that complies with local legislation if a DBD donor
ABO compatibility with the recipient
Serologies (Tissue types compatible for transplantation)
Supplies – tubing for preservation solution, preservation solutions, sternal saws, surgical equipment, bronchoscope, ice, saline, bags for organs, transport devices and organs
Any new information about the donor's history since acceptance of any changes in the donor since acceptance to arrival at the procurement center

Table 3.
Donor procurement checklist [37, 38].

bronchoalveolar lavage. Any bronchial abnormalities or notable pathological findings, such as a lesion suspicious for malignancy, are promptly communicated to the transplant team. These factors may impact the decision regarding the acceptance of the lungs.

7.1.2 Intraoperative assessment of the lungs

The subsequent phase in evaluating a donor involves performing a median sternotomy, which entails surgically exposing the heart and lungs by creating a sizable opening in both pleural spaces. The lungs undergo assessment through visual inspection and palpation to detect masses, bullae, and nodules, and to evaluate for edema, consolidations, or contusions. All identified nodules will have a biopsy to rule out malignancy [36]. Patients who are donors commonly exhibit basal atelectasis due to prolonged mechanical ventilation. To address this, recruitment maneuvers are employed, including lung inflations using a Valsalva technique (air pressure around 20–25 cm H_2O) and gentle expansion of the atelectatic regions. Typically, pulmonary vein gas analysis from all veins is required at FIO2 100% and PEEP of 5–7. Visceral pleural injury is not usually accepted because of risk of lung deflation during transportation and air leak during the surgical implantation [39].

7.2 Donors after cardiocirculatory death (DCD)

Donation after circulatory death (DCD) has the potential to increase the pool of lungs available for transplantation. DCD donors are individuals whose organs are retrieved after cardiac arrest [39]. The established criteria for death involve permanent cessation of both respiration and ventilation [39]. The Maastricht classification identifies four types of DCD donors (I-IV), the first two categories are uncontrolled deaths (uDCD), and the last two are controlled death categories, (cDCD III and IV). See **Table 4**.

Category III donors (cDCD) are preferred in DCD because the patient is in hospital and the process of withdrawal, cardiac arrest, and lung retrieval can be planned and controlled. The duration of warm ischemic time (WIT) for DCD donor lungs has been a subject of debate. Some authors consider that WIT starts when the BP < 50 mm Hg and ends with the onset of pulmonary artery flush [39]. The consensus among most centers is that lungs remain viable for LT within a window of 60 to 90 minutes after circulatory arrest [39]. Donor selection criteria for cDCD are like DBD and extended criteria;

Category	Description	Condition
I	Dead on arrival "in the field"	uncontrolled
II	Unsuccessful resuscitation	uncontrolled
III	Anticipated circulatory arrest	controlled
IV	Circulatory arrest in a patient previously declared brain-dead	controlled
V	Euthanasia or Medical Assistance in Dying (MAID) in hospital	controlled

Table 4.
Donation after cardiac death: Maastricht categories [35].

age > 65 years old, smoking history>20 packs/years, abnormal chest X-Ray, and can be applied to cDCD equally well. The unique aspect of DCD lung retrieval involves conducting bronchoscopy and obtaining arterial gas samples before donor's death. The bronchoscopy can be done in the theater after the reintubation of the airway.

7.3 Living donor lobar lung transplantation (LDLLT)

LDLLT serves as a viable alternative to the traditional lung donation methods (from DBD or DCD donors), particularly in critical situations where a patient may not survive long enough to receive a lung from a DBD or DCD donor. Originally designed for pediatric cystic fibrosis patients, this procedure can now be employed for various conditions like restrictive, obstructive, infectious, or vascular lung disease. Due to its complexity, requiring two living donors, it is typically reserved for centers with expertise in this field [40, 41].

8. Organ procurement and preservation

8.1 Lung procurement technique in DBD donors

The surgical procedure involves two primary steps: preliminary dissection and lung cannulation, followed by lung harvesting. The objective of the preliminary dissection is to isolate essential anatomical structures, facilitating the seamless harvest and preservation of the lungs. The dissection initiates with the placements of pericardial stay sutures, followed by separation of superior vena cava from the pulmonary artery (PA). Subsequently, the dissection progresses involving the inferior vena cava (IVC), ligation of azygos vein (AV), and the separation of the aorta from PA [42]. Both pleurae are widely opened, and pulmonary ligaments are divided. Tracheal dissection is approached between aortic arch and SVC and can be done now or later when the lungs are harvested. Cannulation is done after a 4–0 Polypropylene purse-string suture is placed on the pulmonary artery trunk 1.5 cm proximal to the bifurcation and one more on the ascending aorta. Heparin is administered intravenously 400Units/kg. The cannulas are inserted in the PA and aorta and are connected to the lines and de-aired. The preservation solution (Perfadex) is prepared, and infusion tubes are primed. Prostaglandin E 250 ug is injected into the PA trunk. The SVC is tied and IVC is partially transected, and one pool-tip sucker is inserted into IVC to prevent warm blood from abdominal organ perfusion to reach the pericardium and pleural spaces. The left atrium (LA) appendage is cut to vent the left atrium and prevent heart distension.

The surgical strategy for lung harvest differs if both heart and lungs are collected or only the lungs. If both heart and lungs are harvested best option is to open LAA and insert a pool-tip sucker into the LA. The Waterston interatrial groove is dissected, and LA is open, the heart apex is elevated, and an incision is made into LA between the pulmonary veins and coronary sinus anterior to the left pulmonary veins. Next, an aortic clamp is applied on the ascending aorta, and cardiac preservation solution is started followed by the lung preservation solution. In all this time the lungs will be ventilated with low tidal volumes at FIO2 100% [42]. The cold saline is slushed into the chest around the lungs and the heart. Some surgeons avoid using cold saline for lungs because of risk of injury. The next step is heart explanations which are performed by whole IVC transection, LA incision in Waterston's groove, heart is lifted, and a second incision is made in LA between coronary sinus and left pulmonary veins. The right and left LA incisions are connected, and heart is lifted cephalad, and right and left atriotomies the rest of LA is cut on the superior part. Then the SVC is transected, the aorta is cut distally, and the PA is exposed and transected at bifurcation [43].

The excision of the lung block begins by releasing the pulmonary ligaments, making an incision in the posterior pericardium beyond the pulmonary veins to expose the esophagus (**Figure 1**).

The esophagus serves as a pivotal anatomical reference point for facilitating lung extraction [43]. Dissection on the right side continues on the anterior surface of the esophagus until reaching and dividing the azygos vein. Similarly, on the left side, dissection follows the esophagus and progresses until the aorta which is divided. Subsequently, the anterior exposure of the trachea involves dividing the innominate artery and preparing it circumferentially. With inflation of the lungs and a brief breath hold the trachea is stapled and divided. The lung block is removed from the chest and submerged in an ice solution. An additional retrograde perfusion of 1 liter Perfadex is administered through the pulmonary veins to flush any potential clots from the pulmonary arteries [43]. One the flushing process results in clear fluid the lungs are typically separated and placed in a sterile plastic bag filled with preservation solution. This bag, along with two more plastic bags filled with ice solution, is utilized to store the lungs in an ice cooler for transportation to the recipient hospital.

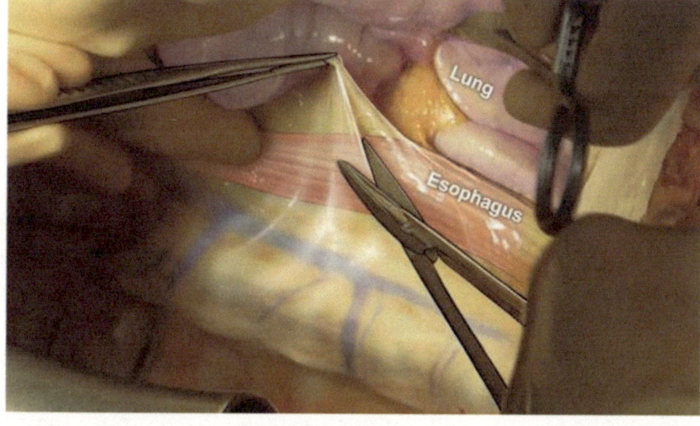

Figure 1.
Dissection of the anterior margin of the esophagus on right and left side [15, 43]. This is an open access article, distributed under the terms of the creative commons attribution non-commercial license https://creativecommons.org/licenses/by-nc/4.0 which permits unrestricted non-commercial use, distribution, and reproduction in any medium, provided the original work is properly cited.

8.2 Lung procurement in DCD donors

Lung procurement in DCD is different from that of DBD donors and the main steps are described below. The procedure begins with a notification to the operating theater to be ready for DCD procurement. Subsequently, a pre-withdrawal meeting convenes, involving all relevant staff. This meeting serves to review the consent details and delineate responsibilities. The withdrawal takes place in either the ICU or the operating room, with inotropic support discontinued and extubation performed [38]. The process of controlled DCD (cDCD) lung retrieval starts with withdrawal from life support if the cardiac arrest occurs in 60–90-minutes intervals [42]. If the cardiac arrest happens, then death is caused by lack of pulsatility of arterial line with or without electrical activity [38] and heparin can be given at this stage (or before the cardiac arrest). There is a "no touch" period of usually 2–5 minutes. If the heparin was administered after death certified, 20 chest compressions are necessary for heparin to circulate in the body. The patient is moved to the operating theater where the surgical team is ready for surgery. The endotracheal tube either remains in place or is removed and the patient is reintubated in theater and a single breath is given until the perfusion solution is started and aorta is clamped to avoid cerebral perfusion resuscitation. [38, 42]. Median sternotomy is performed, and the pulmonary artery is cannulated, Prostaglandin E1 500 micrograms and Perfadex solution are perfused into the lungs (50–70 ml/kg) antegrade and retrograde. The bronchoscopy can be done at this stage by one of the surgeons or anesthesiologists. The left atrial appendage is open for draining the perfusion solution and the lungs are ventilated. The pleural spaces are open, cold saline is infused and the lungs are inspected. The heart is explanted, and the lungs are removed from the chest, with same technique as in DBD previously presented, retrograde flushing is performed packing and storage as in DBD, and are transported to the recipient hospital [42]. If the lungs are borderline, they will be removed en bloc (without separation) and sent to the main hospital for *ex vivo* perfusion (EVLP) to be assessed and repaired. The decision for LT will be delayed at the end of the EVLP [42].

8.3 *Ex vivo* lung perfusion (EVLP)

EVLP is a technique aimed at increasing the number of lung transplants by assessing and repairing borderline organs. To accomplish this the lungs are ventilated and perfused outside the body. It is well-known that lungs suffer many injuries during the harvesting time, because of warm ischemia secondarily to the type of donation (DCD or DBD) or because of the donor pathology itself, smoking, chest contusion, aspiration, pneumonia, etc. *Ex vivo* lung perfusion (EVLP) provides critical insights into lung function and can potentially address some deficiencies, ultimately rendering the organ suitable for transplantation. The rationale behind EVLP lies in the advantages of maintaining normal lung temperature, providing oxygen and nutrients, and allowing real-time assessment and rehabilitation of the lungs.

EVLP employs a centrifugal pump for perfusion and follows a lung protective strategy using low tidal volumes for ventilation. Various protocols exist for EVLP, the Toronto protocol being widely adopted due to its extensive experience [44]. The Toronto protocol involves using acellular perfusate, a closed circuit maintaining positive left atrial pressure, and a low perfusion flow. The process includes specific steps such as connecting the lung graft to the perfusion system, initiating perfusion with solution, and gradually warming the lungs while employing protective ventilation strategies. Throughout the EVLP procedure, assessment is conducted regularly, including arterial gas analysis, pressure measurements, compliance checks, and solution loss. Additionally, X-rays and bronchoscopies are performed. Upon completion, the lungs are cooled, prepared according to the standard preservation protocols, and if deemed suitable, are readied for transplantation in the operating suite. A recent study reaffirmed that when evaluating lung quality, compliance, and airway pressures carry greater significance than oxygenation capacity. There are no differences in CLAD between the LT post-EVLP group and non-EVLP LT [45].

9. Lung transplantation-surgical aspects

There are two main procedures routinely used in COPD, Single Lung Transplantation (SLT) and Double Lung Transplantation (DLT). In special circumstances, living donor lobar lung transplantation (LDLLT) can be a solution for small chest recipients or children where the chance to get an adult donor of the same size is low. Choice of procedure. Single lung transplantation and double lung transplantation are both recommended in patients with severe COPD, but for A1AT DLT is the procedure recommended.

9.1 Single lung transplantation (SLT)-surgical technique

Single lung transplantation is a very useful procedure for end-stage COPD because technically easier, less time-consuming, and less blood loss and intraoperative complications.

9.1.1 Position

The patient is placed in a lateral decubitus or supine position for either postero-lateral or anterolateral thoracotomy. Preparations for ECMO involve marking the femoral artery pulsations on both sides of the inguinal areas. The airway is intubated with a left-sided double-lumen tube or single-lumen tube in smaller patients with a blocker to permit single lung ventilation. Typically, the routine requirements for lung transplantation include the use of an autologous blood recovery system like cell saver, along with a Swan Ganz catheter for monitoring pulmonary artery pressure. Additionally, a deep venous catheter is commonly inserted into a jugular vein [46].

9.1.2 Approach

The incision is usually in the fifth postero-lateral intercostal space or 4th intercostal space for anterolateral thoracotomy.

9.1.3 Pneumonectomy

At this point one-lung ventilation takes place, and cardiac assistance devices such as ECMO or cardiopulmonary bypass (CPB) are employed in the event of hypoxia or hemodynamic instability. If the patient has severe pulmonary hypertension is better to start cardiac assistance before one-lung ventilation [47]. The initial stage is pneumonectomy which begins by accessing the pleural space, releasing the adhesions between the lung and pleura. The electrocautery is used for cutting the adhesions and achieving hemostasis. Afterward, the pulmonary veins are dissected and separated using a stapler prior to the initial division, followed by the dissection and section of the pulmonary artery beyond the first lobar branch. Then the bronchus is transected before the origin of the upper lobe branch, facilitating the removal of the lung from the chest. The peri bronchial tissue may be preserved to avoid the risk of ischemic damage. Hemostasis can be attained by identifying and halting bleeding from bronchial arteries.

9.1.4 Hilar preparation

Following lung removal, the stumps of bronchus and pulmonary vessels are identified and meticulously dissected to enhance their length and mobility. The peri bronchial tissue undergoes careful dissection, with a partial preservation approach aimed to prevent bronchial ischemia. This method ensures that bleeding from bronchial arteries or mediastinal tissue can be promptly addressed before proceeding to the anastomosis.

9.1.5 Donor lung preparation

The donor lung preparation takes place on the back table after removal from the ice box and involves examining the pulmonary artery, pulmonary veins, and bronchus integrity and trimming out the excessive surrounding tissue. In cases where the atrial cuff is insufficiently long and lacks tissue around pulmonary veins, an autologous pericardium patch can be used for enlargement [47]. The size of pulmonary artery is meticulously assessed, and if it is found to be excessively long, adjustments are made to prevent kinking and thrombosis of the anastomosis. The assessment of lung size involves comparing the chest dimensions usually by total lung capacity (predicted and actual). If the lung is deemed excessively large, a reduction surgery on the back table may be considered [47], or if considered can be oversized on purpose. Subsequently, the bronchus is sectioned, the lung is deflated, and is introduced in the chest for implantation.

9.1.6 Lung implantation

The process of lung implantation initiates with bronchial anastomosis, followed by the connection of the pulmonary artery and the left atrial cuff, encompassing the pulmonary veins [46].

9.1.7 Bronchial anastomosis

Bronchial anastomosis is the first anastomosis and requires meticulous attention due to the elevated risk of complications associated with ischemia or technical errors. The bronchus length is carefully assessed and divided by a scalpel, approximately 1 cartilage before the secondary carina, ensuring it's as short as feasible without raising the risk of dehiscence. Various techniques have been devised for bronchial anastomosis. The first technique involves a continuous running suture around the entire circumference using a 4/0 polydioxanone suture.

Another technique largely used employs a posterior running suture on the membranous part of the bronchus, completed by interrupted stitches on the anterior cartilaginous part (see **Figure 2**). This technique is used by most surgeons because gives less complications. If there is a mismatch between the bronchi a telescopic suture is used by taking smaller bites on the donor aiming to fit the donor bronchus

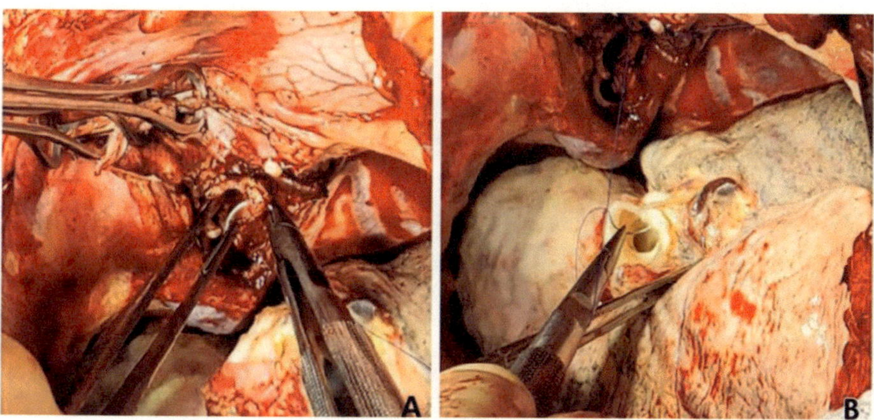

Figure 2.
Right bronchial anastomosis (A) First suture outside-in on recipient at membranous-cartilaginous part (B) Same suture inside-out in the donor bronchus [48]. Open access this article is licensed under a creative commons attribution 4.0 international license, which permits use, sharing, adaptation, distribution and reproduction in any medium or format, as long as you give appropriate credit to the original author(s) and the source, provide a link to the creative commons license, and indicate if changes were made. The images or other third party material in this article are included in the article's creative commons license, unless indicated otherwise in a credit line to the material. If material is not included in the article's creative commons license and your intended use is not permitted by statutory regulation or exceeds the permitted use, you will need to obtain permission directly from the copyright holder. To view a copy of this license, visit http://creativecommons.org/licenses/by/4.0/.

into the recipient [48]. Afterward, an air leak test is performed, and the anastomosis integrity is checked by intraoperative bronchoscopy.

9.1.8 The pulmonary artery anastomosis

The arterial anastomosis is the second anastomosis and initiates with the application of a clamp at the proximal site of PA followed by the careful adjustment of the two arterial stumps. Typically, a continuous 5.0 polypropylene suture is used, starting at the posterior wall, and progressing to the anterior wall (see **Figure 3**). The clamp is left in place until the left atrial (LA) anastomosis is completed facilitating de-airing of the lung [46].

9.1.9 Left atrial anastomosis

The final anastomosis, involving the left atrium (LA) commences with careful application of a Satinski clamp to ensure uninterrupted coronary artery flow and prevent hemodynamic instability. The recipient LA stump is incised, creating two openings that are subsequently joined to form a single anastomotic site. Both LA openings are meticulously readjusted by trimming the excess tissue, and the LA anastomosis is carried out using a single continuous non-resorbable polypropylene 4.0 suture [46]. Some surgeons opt for an everting technique, to prevent muscular tissue from reaching the LA cavity and increasing the thrombotic risk (**Figure 4**).

9.1.10 Lung reperfusion

The lung reperfusion goal is de-airing the lung vasculature to avoid brain and coronary artery embolism. Two methods are available: retrograde flush or antegrade

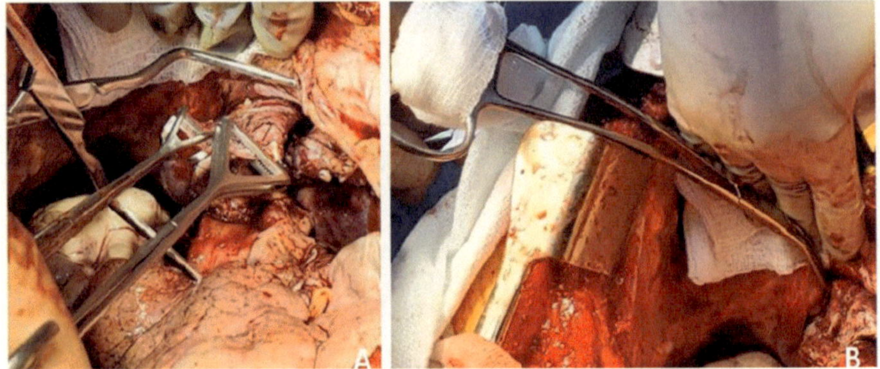

Figure 3.
(A) Right pulmonary artery anastomosis-Duval clamp and Babcock forceps to hold the PA stump. (B) Clamp is wrapped and fixed to the drape followed by artery opening and preparation for anastomosis [48].

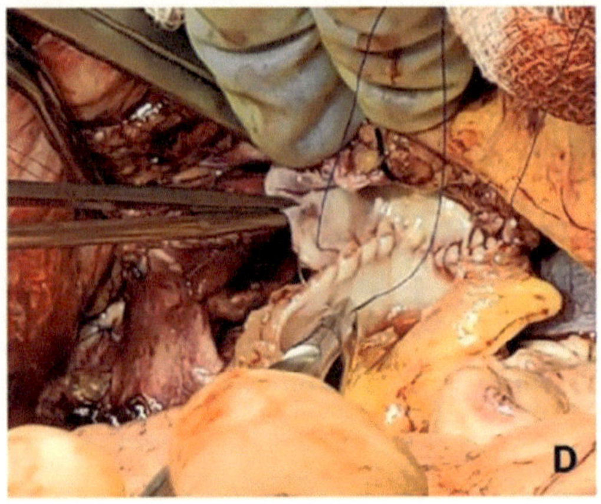

Figure 4.
See the intima-to-intima suture of LA anastomosis. The left atrial anastomosis posterior wall suture between donor and recipient LA [48].

flush, both of which should be completed to achieve optimal results. The retrograde flush involves opening the atrial clamp while keeping the arterial clamp in place coupled with gentle lung ventilation. Conversely, the antegrade flush begins by slowly releasing the pulmonary artery (PA) clamp, keeping the left atrium (LA) clamp closed, and ultimately releasing the atrial clamp [46].

9.1.11 Thoracotomy closure

Following lung implantation and reperfusion, two pleural drains are inserted, and the thoracotomy is closed in anatomical layers. In cases where the sternum was cut to improve exposure during the procedure, the sternal edges will be reapproximated using sternal wires [46].

9.2 Double lung transplantation-surgical technique

Usually, the patient is in supine position, and the chest, abdomen, and legs are prepared for surgery. The site of both femoral arteries is identified and pointed by a marking pen. The most used incision for double lung transplantation (DLT) involves a bilateral anterolateral thoracotomy combined with sternotomy (clamshell incision). This approach offers the best exposure for both lungs and facilities access to the pericardium, especially when using veno- arterial extracorporeal membrane oxygenation (ECMO). Alternatively, bilateral anterolateral thoracotomies without sternal cuts can be used to avoid sternal involvement. However, this method provides less exposure. In rare cases requiring cardiopulmonary bypass, median sternotomy can be utilized. DLT involves sequential explanting and implanting of the new lungs, starting with the more severely affected lung and then proceeding to the other. Anesthesia uses a double-lumen ventilation endotracheal tube for selective ventilation, along with transesophageal echocardiography and intraoperative bronchoscopy during surgery. Following the clamshell incision, and sternal cut specific attention is paid to dividing both internal mammary arteries, and then the pleural cavity is opened. The surgery progresses with the explant of the first lung by separating pleural adhesions and division of the inferior pulmonary ligament. Preservation of the phrenic nerve may be considered. Tapes are used to encircle the pulmonary veins and arteries, which are then cut by stapler. The bronchus is subsequently divided with a scalpel, and meticulous hemostasis of the bronchial arteries is necessary to prevent bleeding which becomes difficult to control once the new lung is in situ [35]. The implanting of the first lung uses the techniques described in SLT surgical procedure. The lung more severely affected by disease is prioritized for transplantation. Once the first lung is implanted, it is reperfused and the decision to use the Extracorporeal Membrane Oxygenation (ECMO) or CPB depends on any alterations in hemodynamics or oxygenation. Some experts advocate for routine CPB usage in DLT to prevent overperfusion of one lung during the implantation of the second, which can elevate the risk of post-transplantation Graft Dysfunction (PGD). Recent years have seen successful utilization of ECMO in these scenarios, offering a lower risk of bleeding compared with CPB, a reduced systemic inflammatory response, and a low transfusion rate [35, 47]. The implantation process for the second lung follows a similar protocol, commencing with pneumonectomy. Subsequently, the lung is implanted, and a bronchoscopy is conducted to verify the patency of the bronchial tree.

9.3 Living donor lung transplantation (LDLLT)

LDLLT consists of a right lower lobectomy from right-side donor, a left lower lobectomy from a left-side donor, and bilateral lobar implantation for the recipient [49]. The procedure is very complex and is recommended to be done in centers with experience in the field. It addresses very sick patients cohort which have no time to wait for a DBD or DCD donor. Size matching is very important as only two lobes are implanted and both functional and anatomical matching are used for evaluation. The procedure needs three operating rooms and four surgical teams, for right-side donor, left-side donor, back table team, and recipient team. The LDLLT is done with ECMO or Cardiopulmonary bypass (CPB). The main steps of the procedure are clamshell incision with sternal division, followed by ECMO placement, right pneumonectomy, right graft implantation and reperfusion, left pneumonectomy followed by left graft implantation and reperfusion, weaning the ECMO, and chest closure. After harvesting the lobes are flushed with a preservation solution before implantation [49].

10. Early surgical complications after lung transplantation

Primary surgical complications following lung transplantation can be categorized into airway, vascular, and additional complications, such as pleural, size mismatch, phrenic nerve palsy, or wound-related problems. Primary graft dysfunction frequently occurs following LT, while other complications such as acute and chronic allograft rejection are not referred to in the present chapter.

10.1 Airway complications

Arise because of bronchial ischemia, attributed to the division of bronchial arteries responsible for vascularizing the bronchus, the blood supply is assured by retrograde flow from the pulmonary artery. This encompasses conditions such as ischemia, necrosis, stenosis, dehiscence, and malacia [50]. Typically, necrosis either resolves spontaneously or progresses to dehiscence, which can be addressed through stent implantation. In severe instances, surgical repair becomes imperative. Following re-anastomosis vascularized flaps from intercostal muscle, or omentum can be employed to facilitate recovery. Stenosis is a common complication that often requires balloon dilatation or argon plasma therapy for resolution [50].

10.2 Vascular complications

Primary vascular complications are bleeding, stenosis of the anastomosis, thrombosis of PA or pulmonary veins, and kinking. Bleeding at the anastomosis usually requires reinforcement, although this may elevate the risk of stenosis. If the bleeding proves uncontrollable, it may be necessary to redo the anastomosis. Kinking occurs when the two arterial stumps are excessively long, potentially leading to thrombosis (**Figure 5**).

Treatment typically involves anticoagulation and insertion of a stent. Pleural complications are effusion, pneumothorax, empyema or chylothorax. Post-lung transplantation pneumothorax is a relatively common occurrence attributed to lung mismatch, air leak resulting from bronchial anastomotic dehiscence, or parenchymal issues. Typically, resolution is achieved through the appropriate management of chest drains [51].

10.3 Primary graft dysfunction (PGD)

PGD stands out as a prevalent cause of early morbidity in lung transplantation, with an incidence of 30% [50]. It manifests through hypoxia and radiologic opacities within the initial 72 hours following surgery (**Figure 6**). Bronchoscopy is used in these cases to evaluate the bronchial anastomosis and to obtain samples for microbiology [51].

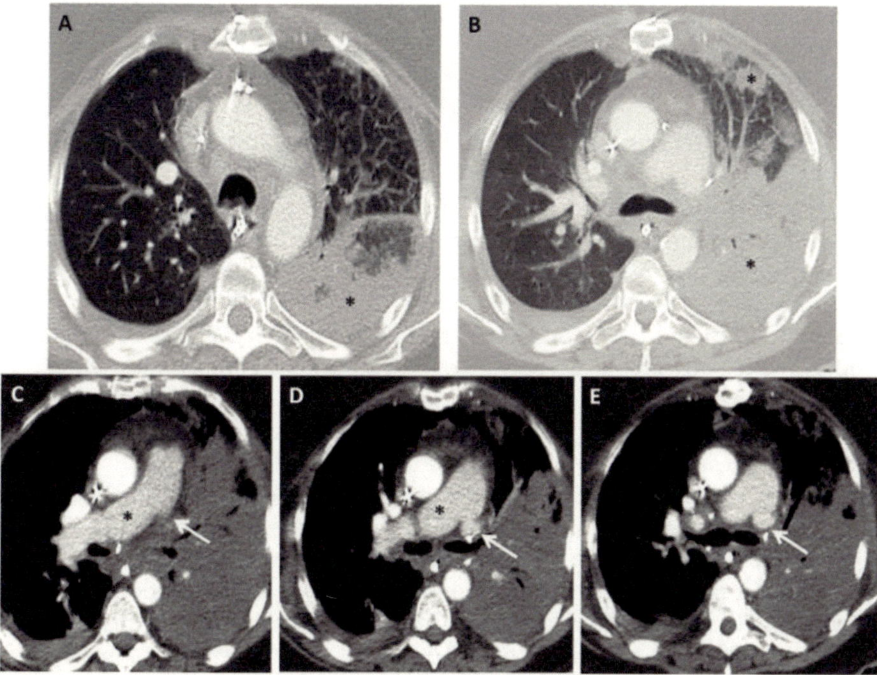

Figure 5.
Left pulmonary artery anastomotic occlusion post-lung transplantation [51]. The author(s).2019 open access this article is distributed under the terms of the creative common international license (https://creativecommons.org/license/by/4.0), which permits unrestricted use, distribution, and reproduction in any medium, provided you give appropriate credit to the original author(s) and the source, provide a link to the creative commons license, and indicate if changes are made.

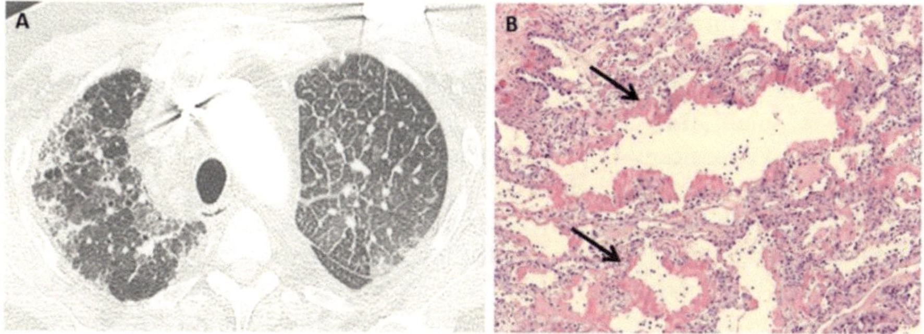

Figure 6.
Primary graft dysfunction [51]. Axial CT images show smooth interlobular septal thickening with ground-glass opacities in the transplanted left lung [22]. The author(s).2019 open access this article is distributed under the terms of the creative common international license (https://creativecommons.org/license/by/4.0), which permits unrestricted use, distribution, and reproduction in any medium, provided you give appropriate credit to the original author(s) and the source, provide a link to the creative commons license, and indicate if changes are made primary graft dysfunction: Imaging and transbronchial biopsy findings. Axial CT images show smooth interlobular thickening with ground-glass opacities in the transplanted left lung.

10.4 Other complications

Encompasses wound dehiscence, diaphragmatic palsy, or heart compression leading to pulmonary edema, particularly in double lung transplantation with oversized lungs. Addressing the latter complication may require temporary maintenance of an open chest cavity.

11. Early and long-term outcomes in lung transplantation for COPD

The success of lung transplantation (LT) for chronic obstructive pulmonary disease (COPD) is highly dependent on timing of the procedure. Optimal timing is critical, as undergoing LT too early may decrease survival rates, while waiting too long can lead to an increased mortality rate on the waiting list. While age itself does not impose a limitation on LT, it's noteworthy that there is a 20% increase in patients aged over 60. However, advancing age may introduce additional comorbidities, potentially contributing to a decrease in 10-year survival rates [33]. The extended donor lung criteria have demonstrated that including heavy smokers as donors does not adversely impact long-term survival. Moreover, individuals positive for hepatitis B and C can be considered viable donors for lung transplantation. In some cases, nonmelanoma skin cancer donors may not pose a significant barrier to lung transplantation and LT might be possible in pulmonary embolism if emboli are well-managed [33]. The utilization of controlled deceased circulatory death donors (cDCD) has led to a donation rate surge of 20–50% in certain countries, whether employing *ex vivo* lung perfusion (EVLP) or not. Effective utilization of EVLP proved advantageous for assessing and repairing lungs, enabling a secure extension of preservation time by over 12 hours without adversely impacting long-term survival.

The A1AT cohort demonstrated a superior median survival compared to the COPD cohort (6.4 vs. 5.5 years) [52]. However, it's worth noting that the A1AT cohort had a younger age at the time of transplant (51.9 vs. 59.7), which may explain the improved survival. In terms of long-term survival, the A1AT cohort exhibited a 43% survival rate, while the COPD cohort showed a lower survival rate of 23% [52]. In the initial year post-LT, the primary causes of death were infection and graft failure. However, in the long term, chronic lung allograft dysfunction (CLAD) emerged as the predominant cause of mortality [53]. Concerning double-lung transplantation (DLT) versus single lung transplantation (SLT), COPD stands out as the primary indication for SLT, with no observed enhancement in long-term survival for DLT [53]. When comparing lung transplantation in controlled donation after circulatory death (DCD) with donation after brain death (DBD), the one-year survival rates were 97 versus 90%, and at 5-year mark, the rates were 90 versus 61% [38]. Long-term survival rates for living donor lobar lung transplantation (LDLLT) in centers with extensive expertise in the field are 80% at 5 years, 72.6% at 10 years, and 61.7% at 15 years [54]. According to Verleden et al. [55] after the ISHLT report, the one-year survival post-lung transplantation (LT) is reported at 87%. The overall 5-year survival rate is 71%, with DLT exhibiting a more favorable outcome at 74% compared to 61% for SLT. Delving into 5-year mortality rates, chronic obstructive pulmonary disease (COPD) records 70.4%, while idiopathic pulmonary fibrosis (IPF) stands at 67%. Notably, the median survival for COPD and A1AT is significantly higher at 7.9 years, surpassing COPD without A1AT at 6.2 years [55]. In a study conducted by Gulack BC [56], examining 9569 patients of whom 14.6% were diagnosed with A1AT, unadjusted comparisons for SLT patients' characteristics, revealed that individuals with A1AT tend to be younger and less prone to smoking, hypertension, or diabetes. When unadjusted outcomes were compared between A1AT and COPD, there were statistically significant findings indicating more airway dehiscence and higher likelihood of rejection in the A1AT group compared with COPD alone. The same author [56] in unadjusted comparisons involving DLT for A1AT, found a higher probability of recipients being younger and less likely to be female. Initial outcomes suggested a higher incidence of airway dehiscence and rejection compared to cases involving COPD only. Notably, the total hospital stay tended to be significantly shorter than COPD cohort.

12. Conclusions

Lung transplantation becomes necessary for COPD patients in advanced stages characterized by diminished quality of life, limited life expectancy, and the presence of difficult medical choices.

Evidence support the notion that single lung transplantation is not inferior to double-lung transplantation. Both procedures have now well-defined indications, with individuals with A1AT deficiency considered candidates for DLT and those with emphysema eligible for either SLT or DLT.

Technical factors play a crucial role in the choice between single-lung transplantation (SLT) and double-lung transplantation (DLT). SLT offers the benefit of shorter procedures and fewer intraoperative complications, whereas DLT tends to be longer with a higher likelihood of utilizing blood products or additional devices like ECMO, adding to the overall complexity. Studies have shown that early mortality rates are higher in DLT compared with SLT; however long-term survival, overall, is slightly better with DLT. DLT has another benefit as it can be employed in cases involving marginal donors, where utilizing a single lung is not practical, but employing two lungs is more suitable for ensuring optimal overall function [57]. Lung transplantation for emphysema poses a complexity due to the intricate task of matching the appropriate organ with the suitable recipient at the optimal time.

Author details

Alina Ligia Cornea[1*], Seamus Linnane[2], Peter Riddell[3], Diana Parau[4] and Alexandru Mihai Cornea[3]

1 Beacon Hospital Dublin, Ireland

2 Beacon Hospital Dublin, University College Dublin, Ireland

3 Mater Misericordiae University Hospital, Dublin, Ireland

4 Carol Davila University of Medicine, Romania

*Address all correspondence to: allcornea@yahoo.com

References

[1] Son J, Shin C. Indications for lung transplantation and patient selection. Journal of Chest Surgery. 2022;**55**(4):255-264

[2] Christenson SA, Smith BM, Bafadhel M, Putcha N. Chronic obstructive pulmonary disease. The Lancet. 2022;**399**(10342):2227-2242

[3] Yang IA, Jenkins CR, Salvi SS. Chronic obstructive pulmonary disease in never-smokers: Risk factors, pathogenesis, and implications for prevention and treatment. The Lancet Respiratory Medicine. 2022;**10**(5):497-511

[4] Safiri S, Carson-Chahhoud K, Noori M, Nejadghaderi SA, Sullman MJM, Heris JA, et al. Burden of chronic obstructive pulmonary disease and its attributable risk factors in 204 countries and territories, 1990-2019: Results from the global burden of disease study 2019. BMJ. 2022;**378**:e069679

[5] Carroll TP, O'Connor CA, Floyd O, McPartlin J, Kelleher DP, O'Brien G, et al. The prevalence of alpha-1 antitrypsin deficiency in Ireland. Respiratory Research. 2011;**12**(1):91

[6] Lachaux A, Dumortier J. Hepatic involvement in hereditary alpha-1-antitrypsin deficiency. Revue des Maladies Respiratoires. 2014;**31**(4):357-364

[7] Gooptu B, Ekeowa UI, Lomas DA. Mechanisms of emphysema in α1-antitrypsin deficiency: Molecular and cellular insights. The European Respiratory Journal. 2009;**34**(2):475-488

[8] Hiller AM, Piitulainen E, Tanash H. The clinical course of severe Alpha-1-antitrypsin deficiency in patients identified by screening. International Journal of Chronic Obstructive Pulmonary Disease. 2022;**17**:43-52

[9] Miravitlles M, Dirksen A, Ferrarotti I, Koblizek V, Lange P, Mahadeva R, et al. European Respiratory Society statement: Diagnosis and treatment of pulmonary disease in α(1)- antitrypsin deficiency. The European Respiratory Journal. 2017;**50**(5):1700610

[10] Giacoboni D, Barrecheguren M, Esquinas C, Rodríguez E, Berastegui C, López-Meseguer M, et al. Characteristics of candidates for lung transplantation due to chronic obstructive pulmonary disease and alpha-1 antitrypsin deficiency emphysema. Archivos de Bronconeumología. 2015;**51**(8):379-383

[11] Riley L, Lascano J. Clinical outcomes and survival following lung transplantation in patients with Alpha-1 antitrypsin deficiency. Respiratory Medicine. 2020;**172**:106145

[12] Zamora MR, Ataya A. Lung and liver transplantation in patients with alpha-1 antitrypsin deficiency. Therapeutic Advances in Chronic Disease. 2021;**12** (Suppl.):20406223211002988

[13] Young AL, Bragman FJS, Rangelov B, Han MK, Galbán CJ, Lynch DA, et al. Disease progression Modeling in chronic obstructive pulmonary disease. American Journal of Respiratory and Critical Care Medicine. 2020;**201**(3):294-302

[14] Celli BR, Cote CG, Marin JM, Casanova C, Montes de Oca M, Mendez RA, et al. The body- mass index, airflow obstruction, dyspnea, and exercise capacity index in chronic obstructive pulmonary disease. The New England Journal of Medicine. 2004;**350**(10):1005-1012

[15] Pirard L, Marchand E. Reassessing the BODE score as a criterion for listing COPD patients for lung transplantation.

International Journal of Chronic Obstructive Pulmonary Disease. 2018;**13**:3963-3970

[16] Daher A, Dreher M. The bidirectional relationship between chronic obstructive pulmonary disease and coronary artery disease. Herz. 2020;**45**(2):110-117

[17] Barnes PJ, Celli BR. Systemic manifestations and comorbidities of COPD. The European Respiratory Journal. 2009;**33**(5):1165-1185

[18] Santambrogio L, Tarsia P, Mendogni P, Tosi D. Transplant options for end stage chronic obstructive pulmonary disease in the context of multidisciplinary treatments. Journal of Thoracic Disease. 2018;**10**(Suppl. 27):S3356-S3365

[19] Ashraf O, Disilvio B, Young M, Ghosh S, Cheema T. Surgical interventions for COPD. Critical Care Nursing Quarterly. 2021;**44**(1):49-60

[20] Slama A, Ceulemans LJ, Hedderich C, Boehm PM, Van Slambrouck J, Schwarz S, et al. Lung volume reduction followed by lung transplantation in emphysema-a Multicenter matched analysis. Transplant International: Official Journal of the European Society for Organ Transplantation. 2022;**35**:10048

[21] Laupacis A, Sackett DL, Roberts RS. An assessment of clinically useful measures of the consequences of treatment. The New England Journal of Medicine. 1988;**318**(26):1728-1733

[22] Leard LE, Holm AM, Valapour M, Glanville AR, Attawar S, Aversa M, et al. Consensus document for the selection of lung transplant candidates: An update from the international society for heart and lung transplantation. The Journal of Heart and Lung Transplantation: The Official Publication of the International Society for Heart Transplantation. 2021;**40**(11):1349-1379

[23] Weill D, Benden C, Corris PA, Dark JH, Davis RD, Keshavjee S, et al. A consensus document for the selection of lung transplant candidates: 2014-an update from the pulmonary transplantation Council of the International Society for heart and lung transplantation. The Journal of Heart and Lung Transplantation: The Official Publication of the International Society for Heart Transplantation. 2015;**34**(1):1-15

[24] Inci I, Schuurmans M, Ehrsam J, Schneiter D, Hillinger S, Jungraithmayr W, et al. Lung transplantation for emphysema: Impact of age on short- and long-term survival. European Journal of Cardio-thoracic Surgery: Official Journal of the European Association for Cardio-thoracic Surgery. 2015;**48**(6):906-909

[25] Mosher CL, Weber JM, Frankel CW, Neely ML, Palmer SM. Risk factors for mortality in lung transplant recipients aged ≥65 years: A retrospective cohort study of 5,815 patients in the scientific registry of transplant recipients. The Journal of Heart and Lung Transplantation: The Official Publication of the International Society for Heart Transplantation. 2021;**40**(1):42-55

[26] Upala S, Panichsillapakit T, Wijarnpreecha K, Jaruvongvanich V, Sanguankeo A. Underweight and obesity increase the risk of mortality after lung transplantation: A systematic review and meta-analysis. Transplant International: Official Journal of the European Society for Organ Transplantation. 2016;**29**(3):285-296

[27] Bals R, Boyd J, Esposito S, Foronjy R, Hiemstra PS, Jiménez-Ruiz CA, et al. Electronic cigarettes: A task force report from the European Respiratory Society.

The European Respiratory Journal. 2019;**53**(2):1801151

[28] Veit T, Munker D, Leuschner G, Mümmler C, Sisic A, Kauke T, et al. High prevalence of falsely declaring nicotine abstinence in lung transplant candidates. PLoS One. 2020;**15**(6):e0234808

[29] Mekov E, Ilieva V. Machine learning in lung transplantation: Where are we? Presse Médicale. 2022;**51**(4):104140

[30] Barac Y, Silvestri SC, Daneshmand MA, Goldstein JD. Textbook of Transplantation and Mechanical Support for End-Stage Heart and Lung Transplantation. USA: John Wiley & Sons Ltd; 2024. p. 1037

[31] Riddell P, Egan JJ. International donor conversion rates for lung transplantation need to be standardized. The Lancet Respiratory Medicine. 2015;**3**(12):909-911

[32] Vos R, Patterson A, Raemdonck DV. In: LoCicero J III, Feins RH, Colson YL, Gaetano R, editors. Chapter 88, Shield's General Thoracic Surgery. 8th ed. USA: Wolters Kluwer; 2019. pp. 1115-1143. Available from: https://lccn.loc.gov/2017051947

[33] Van der Mark S, Hoek RAS, Hellemons ME. Developments in lung transplantation over the past decade. European Respiratory Review. 2020;**29**:190132. DOI: 10.1183/16000617.0132-2019

[34] Aleyadeh W, Verna EC, Elbeshbeshy H, Sulkowski MS, Smith C, Darling J, et al. Outcomes of early vs late treatment initiation in solid organ transplantation from hepatitis C virus nucleic acid test-positive donors to hepatitis C virus-uninfected recipients: Results from the HCV-TARGET study. American Journal of Transplantation. 2024;**24**:468-478

[35] Lemaitre PH, Tikkanen JM, Mariscal A, Singer LG, Keshavjee S. Lung transplantation. In: Darling GE, Baumgartner WA, Jacobs JP, editors. Pearson's General Thoracic Surgery. USA: STS Cardiothoracic Surgery E-Book. STS 2021. Ebook.sts.org. The Society of Thoracic Surgeons. 2024. Available from: https://ebook.sts.org/sts/index/Pearsons-General-Thoracic/Thoracic; [Accessed: December 2023]

[36] Krishnan P, Saddoughi SAD. Procurement of lungs from brain-death donors. Indian Journal of Thoracic and Cardiovscular Surgery. 2021;**37**(Suppl. 3): S416-S424. DOI: 10.1007-021-01140-1

[37] Loor G, Shumway SJ, McCurry KR, et al. Process improvement in thoracic donor organ procurement: Implementation of a donor assessment checklist. Annals of Thoracic Surgery. 2016;**102**(6):1872-1877

[38] Copeland H, Hayanga JWA, Neyrink A, et al. Donor Heart and Lung Procurement: A Consensus Statement. Elsevier Inc. on Behalf of International Society for Heart and Lung Transplantation. Jun 2020;**39**(6):501-517. DOI: 10.1016/j.healun.2020.03.020

[39] Inci I. Donors after cardiocirculatory death. Journal of Thoracic Disease. 2017;**9**(8):2660-2669. DOI: 10.21037/jtd.2067.07.82

[40] Date H. Current status and problems of lung transplantation in Japan. Journal of Thoracic Disease. 8 Aug 2016;(Suppl. 8):S631-S636. DOI: 10.21037/jtd.2016.06.38

[41] Date H. Living-related lung transplantation. Journal of Thoracic Disease. 2017;**9**(9):3362-3371. DOI: 10.21037/jtd.2017.08.152

[42] Nguyen DC, Loor G, Carrott P, Shafii A. Review of donor and recipient

surgical procedures in lung transplantation. Journal of Thoracic Disease. 2019;**11**(Suppl. 14):S1810-S1816. DOI: 10.21037/jtd.2019.06.31

[43] Yu WS, Son JA. Donor selection, management, and procurement for lung transplantation. Journal of Chest Surgery. 2022;**55**(4):277-282. DOI: 10.5090/jcs.22.068

[44] Watanabe T, Cypel M, Keshavjee S. *Ex vivo* lung perfusion. Journal of Thoracic Disease. 2021;**13**(11):6602-6617. DOI: 10.21037/jtd-2021-23

[45] Wauwer C, Suylen V, Zhang LZ, et al. Is logistically motivated *ex vivo* lung perfusion a good idea? Frontiers in Transplantation. 2022;**1**:12. DOI: 10.3389/frtra.2022.988950

[46] Gust L, D'Journo XB, Briounde G, et al. Single-lung and double-lung transplantation: Techniques and tips. Journal of Thoracic Disease. 2018;**104**(4):2508-2518. DOI: 10.21037/jtd.2018.03.187

[47] Park S, Kim YT. Technical aspects of lung transplantation: General considerations. Journal of Chest Surgery. 2022;**55**(4):301-306. Available from: https://orcid.org/0000-0001-9006-4881

[48] Murala JS, Hanif HM, Peltz M, et al. Lung transplantation: How to do it. Indian Journal of Thoracic and Cardiovascular Surgery. 2021;**37** (Suppl. 3):S454-S475. DOI: 10.1007/s12055-021-01218-w

[49] Date H. Living-donor lobar lung transplantation. The Annals of Thoracic Surgery. 2021;**112**:1055-1058. Available from: https://10.1016/j.athoracsurg.2021.06.0511

[50] Suh JW. Surgical complications affecting the early and late survival rates after lung transplantation. Journal of Chest Surgery. 2022;**55**(4):332-337. Available from: https://orcid.org/0000-0003-0287-0651

[51] Saeedan MB, Mukhopadhyay S, Lane CR, Renapurkar R. Imaging indications and findings of lung transplant draft dysfunction and rejection. Insights into Imaging. 2020;**11**:2. DOI: 10.1186/s13244-019-0822-7

[52] Riley L, Lascano J. Clinical outcomes and survival following lung transplantation in patients with Alha-1 antitrypsin deficiency. Respiratory Medicine. 2020;**172**:106145. DOI: 10.1016/j.rmed.2020.106145

[53] Greer M, Welte T. Chronic obstructive pulmonary disease and lung transplantation. Seminars in Respiratory and Critical Care Medicine. 2020. DOI: 10.1055/s-0040-1714250

[54] Date H. Living-donor lung transplantation. The Journal of Heart and Lung Transplantation. Article in press. 2023. DOI: 10.j.healun.2023.09.006

[55] Verleden GM, Gottlieb J. Lung transplantation for COPD and emphysema. European Respiratory Review. 2023;**32**:220116. DOI: 10.1183/16000617.0116-2022

[56] Gulack BC, Mulvihill MS, Ganpathy AM, et al. Survival after lung transplantation in recipients with Alpha-1-antitrypsin deficiency compared of chronic obstructive pulmonary disease: A national cohort study. Transplant International. 2018;**31**(1):45-55. DOI: 10.1111/tri.13038

[57] Weill D, Keshavjee S. Lung transplantation for emphysema: Two lungs or one. The Journal of Heart and Lung Transplantation. 2001;**20**:739-742